The Eight Sacred Responsibilities

A GUIDE FOR FIERY AND FABULOUS WOMEN 50+

THE
EIGHT
SACRED
RESPONSIBILITIES
~ CATHY MINES ~

The Eight Sacred Responsibilities

ISBN 978-1-9995100-0-8 (print)
ISBN 978-1-9995100-1-5 (eBook)

Cover design: Cathy Mines
Book design: Ellie Sipila
Editor & project manager: Kirsten Marion
Don Christensen Sacred Campaign Supporter
Printed in Canada

Reach Yoga Lifestyle.

THE EIGHT SACRED RESPONSIBILITIES

If you have ever pondered what your legacy will be once you leave this gorgeous green planet, know that it will be the example you set by taking Sacred Responsibility for your happiness.

Hell yeah, we are in our prime!

~

Cathy Mines RIHR, CYT
Certified Peace Ambassador, Ally, Pilgrim, Student.

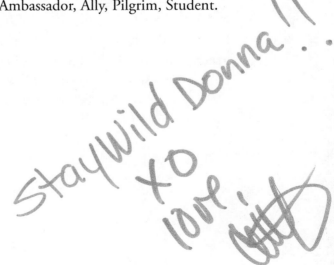

Stay wild Donna!!
XO
love,

LAND ACKNOWLEDGEMENT

I would like to acknowledge that the Reach Yoga office, studio spaces as well as my personal home are situated upon traditional territories of First Nations peoples. The territories include the Huron Wendat Confederacy, Anishinabek Nation, the Haudenosaunee Confederacy, and today, the guardians are the Mississaugas of Scugog (skoo-gog), Hiawatha (hi-ah-wah-tha), Alderville First Nation and the Mississaugas of the New Credit.

The treaty that was signed for this particular parcel of land is collectively referred to as the Williams Treaties of 1923. Prior to contact with Europeans, the sovereign First Nations developed an agreement called "The Dish With One Spoon" to share the land and its resources equally, respectfully and with the understanding of taking only what was needed to live and giving thanks for the bounty of Mother Earth.

May we work together in harmony, may we respect one and other, may we honour the Original Peoples of this land and thank them for caretaking on behalf of future generations and all of us present today. May we learn from their relationship with the natural world.

May we join with the First Peoples in the protection of the natural world.

Thank you.

DEDICATION

Nevertheless, she persisted. This is book is dedicated to women who will not stand down:

Susan B. Anthony, Marguerite Barankitse, Benazir Bhutto, Rosella Bjornson, Nelly Bly, Ruby Bridges, Rachel Carson, Marie Curie, Viola Desmond, Vera Drake, Anne Frank, Rosalind Franklin, Betty Friedan, Margaret Fuller, Ruth Bader Ginsburg, Anita Hill, Mazie Hirono, Katherine Johnson, Henrietta Lacks, Susan LaFlesche, Kahontakwas Diane Longboat, Nellie McClung, Marilyn Monroe, Nadia Murad, Emily Murphy, Emmeline Pankhurst, Rosa Parks, Cecilia Payne, J.K. Rowling, Idola Saint-Jean, Elizabeth Cady Stanton, Gloria Steinem, Emily Howard Stowe, Katherine Switzer, Brandon Teena, Rajani Thiranagama, Marina Triger, Sojourner Truth, Elizabeth Warren, Naomi Weisstein, Mary Wollstonecraft, Malala Yousafzai.

I have only started the list the rest of the space is yours to fill. After all, someone must want Joan of Arc on the list!

TABLE OF CONTENTS

CHAPTER 3. THE THIRD SACRED RESPONSIBILITY: KNOW YOURSELF.

- Living in the present moment. Shining in your authenticity. Unearth the limiting beliefs that hold you back. Knowing what makes your heart sing!

CHAPTER 4. THE FOURTH SACRED RESPONSIBILITY: COLLABORATE.

- Honouring every thread of the tapestry. Observing collaboration in everything.
- Sacred Reciprocity. Trusting yourself.

CHAPTER 5. THE FIFTH SACRED RESPONSIBILITY: HONOUR YOUR INTUITION.

- Respecting your inner wisdom keeper. Following your fine inner compass.
- Release and Nourish. Intimate Relationships.

CHAPTER 6. THE SIXTH SACRED RESPONSIBILITY: CREATE AND PLAY.

- The art of play as a creative process. Keeping it real keeping it fun. Try something new, try something different. Sensuality and living in a turned-on state.

CHAPTER 7. THE SEVENTH SACRED RESPONSIBILITY: RELAX AND CELEBRATE.

- Relaxing as a glowing example of joy, care and kindness.
- Celebrating others. Celebrating yourself. Enjoying growing wiser.
- Ageing gracefully, strong and imbued with story.

CHAPTER 8. THE EIGHTH SACRED RESPONSIBILITY: GRATITUDE.

- Living in a state of gratitude. None of this will reach its full potential without Gratitude.

CHAPTER 9. MAINTAINING OUR CONNECTION AND THE SACRED CIRCLE.

Appendix 1. Chakras 101
Gratitude to My Teachers.
Resources and References.

A LETTER TO THE READER

Welcome to the Movement!

Dear Sacred Readers, you have joined a movement. A movement that is launching the most wonderful and creative project you will ever embark on. This is a project where you are both artist and muse, inspired and the inspiration. A project where your personal heart song joins with women across the globe in harmony. Whether you are singing at the top of your lungs, humming softly or tapping along to your own unique beat, you have joined a movement that starts you on a course of thriving in your third act.

Together we walk the way of the sovereign woman taking sacred responsibility for every aspect of our thoughts, words and actions in a fiery act of defiance over boredom, self-sabotage and old programs.

The Eight Sacred Responsibilities are designed in a way that gives us a protocol to follow, to keep us on track, inspired and in collaboration with all that makes our heart sing. The Responsibilities speak directly to the women who are compelled to rise and shine and want to be part of a plan to make it so. Through each Responsibility we call back the parts of us that are longing to be revived, nurtured and lived to the fullest. We do this by immersing joyfully into sacred responsibility.

Guided by *The Eight Sacred Responsibilities* we re-configure ourselves in ways that honour our highest values and our richest creativity. The protocol gives us a foundation of simple living and by conscious participation, a life well lived begins to unveil itself to us.

Today we commit to the Eight Sacred Responsibilities as we declare to ourselves and each other the following.

Declaration:

Today I open myself fully to living a sacred life, I call in now the people, places and things that lift me up, light me up and hold me up as the accountable, responsible and authentic woman I am here to be. And so it is.

We are calling back the parts of us we have forgotten about, all the parts we set aside long ago. Calling back those parts of us that still flicker in our hearts' like fireflies sparking our memory. Lean in here, ladies, while I whisper in your ear…

You are already fiery and fabulous.

That is what brought you here. What we do now, together, through our practices and community is to enhance our lives in ways that continue to fan our flame. The Eight Sacred Responsibilities are designed to enhance our lives, but make no mistake, you are already fiery and fabulous just by showing up!

The journey of our connection begins here.
May it be a grand collaboration.
In gratitude,

Cathy

INTRODUCTION

The Eight Sacred Responsibilities is a movement of the fiery and fabulous women over fifty who have chosen to make their third act one that includes a future filled with personal standing ovations! Or gracefully seated ones, we get to choose!

This is not only a guide book for the solo sister but a movement that brings women in their "Third Act" together for transformation, collaboration and to hold each other accountable to living an empowered life that honours happiness, creativity and some serious fun!

Fact: we are living 25–30 years longer than the generations before us and that means we have time for an extra full-adult life. This book suggests, and most times insists, we use that time to transform ourselves into the greater version of the passionate, interested and self-knowing women we are here to be, and in that inspire others to rise and shine.

Sacred sisters, it is my absolute pleasure to know you, to stand on this stage with you and to be held accountable by you. Today, together we step into a community of like-hearted, spirited women who join us in awakening to the next act of our lives, our third act.

You will want a companion notebook or journal while on our journey as this book will inspire your creativity as well as your self-reflection and we want to start to collect all of our juicy personal musings as we begin to live a refreshed and empowered life through the Eight Sacred Responsibilities and their practices. When inspiration rises write it down, even if it is just one word circled in purple highlighter. You may find poetry comes to the surface, songs, drawings, and "*Aha!*" moments emerge while uncovering the data stored deep in your cells from your many years of life experience. A Sacred Responsibilities journal has no rules; it evolves as you do. Write, draw, fold corners, spill tea on it, press leaves in it, just let it be as wild as you are!

Defining Sacred Responsibility.
What exactly is a "Sacred Responsibility"? Let me begin with a bit about the word "responsibility". During my teachings of the Sacred Responsibilities I have come across every resistance that I could have imagined and the one I found stood out above the rest is the reaction to the word "responsibility."

It is my hope that together we can re-establish our enthusiasm for responsibility in this life. I wish for us to ignite a passion for the sacredness of human responsibly. Somewhere down the line we have been convinced that responsibility is something to be burdened by. I believe it is something to be elevated by, something to help us thrive, something on which to build a strong foundation. It is our Sacred Responsibility to ignite the fire of our third act.

Let's break it down for ourselves so we have a clear understanding of what it truly means. I have used a combination of Webster's, English Oxford and Collins dictionaries definition of each word to help us to develop an understanding of the foundations of this book and the Eight Sacred Responsibilities: Self-Care, Rise and Shine, Know Yourself, Collaborate, Honour Your Intuition, Create and Play, Relax and Celebrate, Gratitude.

Responsibility: The state of being the person who causes something to happen.

Responsible: a moral obligation or duty; a charge of trust; a thing one is responsible for. The opportunity or ability to act independently and make decisions without authorization.

Adding to the definition of responsibility: our ability to respond. Responsibility to respond in all the ways that increase our life force and vitality. Our ability to choose the response of happiness, love and kindness. And knowing this is a work in progress.

Sacred: Regarded as holy; worthy of or entitled to respect; regarded with reverence. Too important to be changed or interfered with.

In addition to our dictionary definitions we will add: something that is sacred to us and cannot be taken away from us, it is something that is directly connected to the spirit of living an earthbound life while tethered to the great mystery, God, Creator, Great Spirit and all of the names of we know to indicate a force greater then we understand with our minds. The force of love.

From all the above, we can develop a definition of a Sacred Responsibility.

Sacred Responsibility: A highly valued course of action towards personal happiness that is regarded with reverence. A moral obligation to respond to life in ways that increase our life force and vitality.

And before we get our noses out of joint around the word moral, here is how Webster's Dictionary defines moral: "Ethical, good, honest honourable, just, upright, virtuous."

While we are at it, let's look at the definition of obligation, "Accountability, responsibility, agreement, bond, contract."

What we have here is a Sacred Contract for the benefit of our mind, body and soul which we enter into rooted in accountability and wild reverence. Today we drop to our knees in gratitude for the opportunity to reclaim our love for life. It is our Sacred Responsibility to do so.

Taking Sacred Responsibility for Our Happiness

I have always had a deep feeling that we are fully responsible for our own happiness in this life. I have always found myself looking for the fun, joy and connection where ever I am, whatever I am doing. Many times, it is like digging through the rubble of a forgotten city. Women, in particular, have forgotten that we can love and care for those around us without losing ourselves in the process. We are now starting to dig ourselves out from the rubble of meeting everyone else's needs before our own and finding our fabulous selves buried deep, still very much alive! To you sisters who have given all of yourself to others in your life, I welcome you to this fantastic dig site. It is time to get our hands dirty and unearth ourselves. To choose the parts of us that lift us up and leave buried the things that hold us back.

In this book we learn how to reclaim our love of life and steep in it rather than simply seeing sparks of it on occasion. We give ourselves full permission to make self-care a priority in any and all of the ways that suit our state of need. If we are tired, we have permission to sleep. And not just regular old sleep but luxurious sleep! If we are unsure how to solve a problem or balance a situation in our lives we have permission to meditate, breathe and be alone to think from our hearts because we know the power of our alone time. We now give ourselves full permission to live our lives from a perspective of sacred responsibility.

We begin our sacred assignment now with a Magical Moment by breathing together as we dive into this material. Today we, as a collective of seekers from all parts of the globe, deeply honour the simple yet complex gift of our breath. Acknowledging the four parts of our breath in this gentle breathing exercise that helps us re-establish our conscious connection of the breath and body as well as the conscious connection to one another and to the creative source we all come from.

We breathe in through the nose and out through the nose for this practice. Breathe at your natural pace and luxuriate in each of the four parts as you flow through them.

1. Inhale deeply
2. Retain your breath (hold)
3. Exhale deeply
4. Pause (rest here)

Inhale, retain, exhale, pause
Inhale, retain, exhale, pause
Inhale, retain, exhale, pause

Breathe with the intent to connect to this collaborative effort. An effort where we keep these conversations going, expanding our hearts and minds. Taking our lives directly by the hand and walking ourselves straight towards the most authentic expression of who we are in this life and all that we have to offer in this, our third act.

Breathe with your imagination. Imagining as you breathe that we are all connected in this flow of togetherness, support and aliveness.

Now, feel it. Feel it if only for a moment as this is the theme of our practice. Imagine it, feel it, and be it—fiery and fabulous in our third act.

May our breath entrain with the breath of the universe and the breath of each reader as we reclaim the wild and creative connection to our life well lived. This breathing technique is our tether to each other, and our road home to our inner peace. Use this focused breath as part of your everyday practice.

Now you can grab a pen or a highlighter because it's going to get messy! I want you to make notes in this book, fold corners down on the pages that speak to your heart and highlight the heck out of the words that you love. Starting now, go ahead and write today's date, this is your Third Act Conception date. Now calculate the date forward, as eight months from now is your second birthday, your fiery and fabulous Sacred Birthday and we are going to celebrate!

It is on your Sacred Birthday that together we reflect on where we have shifted, changed and created our next chapter in our life well lived. Get ready; our commitment to taking responsibility for our happiness is the fun and messy icing on the cake! (Or for us A-Type personalities you can keep all the icing neatly in your journal.)

Conception Date: _____

My 2nd Birthday: _____

January February March April May June July August
September October November December

Conceive it, believe it, achieve it.

Our Sacred Practices

We women share in the protocol practices with reverence for the potent possibilities that lie dormant within us. We accept our practice with open hearts and open minds in the knowing that these tiny acts of self-care grow quickly into a renewed love of our lives. We know in every cell of our gorgeous being that our practices fill us with the vibrancy of universal life-force.

Ordinary people focus on the outcome, extraordinary people focus on the process. That was the title of a great article by Anthony More that was printed in *Medium Daily Digest* and I loved it! (link to this article is in the back of the book)

Here's to us enjoying focusing on our practice, we all

know there will be an outcome, but how about we enjoy the journey and let the outcomes surprise us!

Now let's get really clear on the formula of our practice so that when we get to our exercises you will know exactly why they work and how they will support your life empowered by Sacred Responsibility. At the end of each Sacred Responsibility chapter you will find three practices:

- One Imagination (Meditation exercise). Representing our Thoughts.
- One Breathing (Life Force exercise). Representing our Words.
- One Physical (Body Care exercise). Representing our Actions.

That is our practice formula. An exercise directly connected to the Sacred Responsibility of the power of our own Thoughts, Words and Actions.

I recommend that as we begin to establish the repetition, habit and flow of our practice and that we cycle through them in order as they appear in the book. Let's keep it simple and attainable as we start to get to know our practice. Prepare to start out with a 1-minute practice daily.

We will make a commitment to ourselves and each other to choose one Imagination, Breathing and Physical practice each day and do it for 1 minute, just to warm ourselves up as we are getting to know ourselves, our bodies and minds and each other. One minute, no excuses, and if you find you are without your book and you are ready to do your practice, but you think you can't remember what to do, go rogue! Use your imagination and move, breathe and imagine yourself in an excellent state of being.

Once you are comfortable with 1 minute, work your way up to 8 minutes of the three exercises for the Sacred Responsibility you are working with. We are always enjoying our exercises and making them a priority each day. We are tapped into the benefits of our breathing, moving, and imagination exercises. We carve out the best time for ourselves personally for our practice. Some of us will Rise and Shine with a morning practice, some of us will Know Ourselves and enjoy an afternoon practice and others will enjoy an evening practice in Gratitude. Personally, I have a mixed schedule and slide into my practices at different times each day, and I work very hard to answer the call of impulse. If I have the impulse to do any of our practice exercises I do my very best to act on it and move my body, breathe and imagine. I am always intrigued by impulse and the creative flow that comes with answering its call.

Once you have built up to an 8-minute daily practice, open yourself up to an expanded practice of 8 minutes for each exercise of imagination, breathing and physical exercise.

Let me do the math for you here, that would mean that our basic practice will, in time, build up to 24 minutes a day. 8 minutes of Imagination/Meditation/Thoughts, 8 minutes of Breathing/Life force/Words and 8 minutes of Physical/Body Care/Action.

Sisters, we have a whole adult life to live together so we have time and a plan! And we most certainly have 8 minutes a day to give 100% focus on our Sacred Responsibility to ourselves. Did you catch that? 100% focus, oh yeah, that's where we are going with this. 100% focus on our practices, on ourselves and cultivating our joy for 8 minutes a day.

We also have audio instructions plus a downloadable PDF of the practices available to you. Enter our Sacred Portal at www.reachyogalifestyle.ca for fun and support. If you have contraindications for any of our physical exercises, do not leave them out of your practice, simply switch them from physical to imagination and do them in your mind. This is a great exercise to play with even if you are incapable of doing them physically. Doing the exercises in your mind will still continue to build new neural pathways.

Repetition of our practices helps us become more conscious of the quality of our thoughts, words and actions. Plus, practice makes perfect they say! Which really means our practice rewires our brain and creates new pathways. Learning makes new connections. This is the basics of brain growth, of neuroplasticity. Our brain will assemble new circuits with our practice. *And* we will enjoy doing it, laying down the circuits of our new third act personality, mind and body!

The idea of our practices having a time limit is simply our way to begin to create new pathways in our brain. We now do something new every day that benefits the sacred health of our mind, body, and heart. As we find ourselves mastering the practices we get creative, we expand our imagination even more, our breath goes to the next level of richness and our connection to the physical becomes more enjoyable and we do the practices for the length of time that feels most natural to each of us.

How will you know when it is time to extend the

number of minutes? First, you will be surprised that the 1-minute or 8, or 24 minutes is up already. And second, you will find yourself in a rhythm of inner peace that is so luxurious and real that you will prefer to hold yourself in this Sacred State for longer. We set up our template, get grounded in it, then fly as high and as far as we desire.

Once we are established in easeful repetition of our exercises, these practices can be done in any order, as often as you like and for as long as you feel good doing them.

The power of our practice is simple.

Our thoughts create our reality, and it is imperative to have an imagination practice rich with healthy ways of thinking and imagining ourselves in our lives. The

Your beliefs become your thoughts. Your thoughts become your words. Your words become your actions. Your actions become your habits. Your habits become your values. Your values become your destiny.

—Gandhi

subconscious mind (from which we are operating 95% of the time) accepts everything we think and tell ourselves as true and it will work outside of our conscious awareness to prove us right. Which is exactly why we have a daily practice of thinking and imagining our life well-lived. We may as well think, imagine and create each day in ways that serve to reduce stress, make us laugh and bring us joy.

The first way we take Sacred Responsibility for ourselves is by luxuriating in the thoughts and feelings that we most desire to experience. We will learn and practice sending "Sacred Packages" forward, look into the sciences that support our practices and you will be pleasantly surprised at the power in the simplicity of our practice.

Throughout our time together reading, connecting and co-creating our third act we are building a practice. A daily practice that is unique to each of us yet modeled by the Eight Sacred Responsibilities.

Self-Care, Rise and Shine, Know Yourself, Collaborate, Honour Your Intuition, Create and Play, Relax and Celebrate and Gratitude. For the record. I never get bored typing them out, and I do not cut and paste The Eight Sacred Responsibilities. Writing or typing them makes me happy and begins to build the foundation of the practice by knowing them not only in my mind, but my heart and in my cells.

I have found what matters most to me at this junction in my life. What has helped me most to find more glimpses of happiness than sorrow, is my practice of these particular things in my life, The Eight Sacred Responsibilities. I enjoy writing them out, I write them in my journal, in my emails, texts, and in the art I create. I sing them, and I say them and when I notice someone naturally doing one of them or talking about one of them I say, "Hey! That is amazing, that's the Sixth Sacred Responsibility: Create and Play!"

An evolved life requires balance. Sometimes you have to cut out one thing to find balance everywhere else.

—Sarah Hepola

In order for me to be the best example, I have made it my life's work to live by these pillars. I work (well really play) with the practices, I teach them, and I look for signs of them manifesting in all ways in my life. I collect stories from others who are also using this practice as a roadmap to a life well-lived, and because I have a road map to follow I am in a continual flow of building resilience, strength and flexibility. This means if, or when, I am hit with a physical or an emotional challenge I have a strong foundation from which to respond. This is what I wish for all of us!

Then and Now. Resiliency and the Sacred Woman
The platform and guidance of the Eight Sacred Responsibilities is our foundation to thrive from in our third act as well as the foundation of our community. A sacred community of women where we can hold each other accountable to living a thriving and fulfilled life.

Together as we walk through the gates of a reclaimed life ready and willing to rise and shine we pause in honour of all our life's experience up until this point. We pause and honour all the experiences that have shaped us, and many times surprised us.

It is often hard to see the strength, purpose or wisdom of things from our past experiences until we get a little space between then and now. You know how hard it is to see the details of something that you hold right up to your nose. But if you hold it at arms-length you begin to see all of it.

This applies to our experiences, too. Putting some distance between us and our experiences in life often reveals the wisdom and the lessons. As we find ourselves here in our third act we have plenty of space and time between so many things we have experienced and where we are now.

I often make this point in my classes that it's Monday

morning and we are all gathered around the proverbial water cooler talking about what we did on our weekends and the conversation inevitably goes something like this.

"Hey, how was your weekend?"

"Great! I ran a half marathon."

"Wow that's impressive. Woot Woot!"

"How about you? How was your weekend?"

"Oh, it was great too! I did a breathing meditation and some barefoot walking in the park."

…crickets…chirp…chirp…

We haven't quite got to the point in society where peaceful practices are seen with equal enthusiasm as highly active practices. But persevere, sisters, we are pioneering souls shining a light on living authentically where both marathons and meditation reside together for the choosing. We continue with our simple practices quietly and sometimes secretly building up our strength and resilience. Our practices teach us how not to leak our energy and in that, prepare us for the marathons of life.

Beginning in the Past
Women in the third act, it is time to move ahead. What we have been doing no longer works. More importantly we are no longer needed to do the same things we have been doing. The things that we have been directing our time and attention towards no longer need us in the same ways that they have in the past and this puts us at a crossroads.

A big part of shifting ourselves fully into the third act of our lives is acknowledging that much of where we gave our attention in our adult lives is no longer necessary to the same extent it was in the past.

We are no longer raising small children at this stage of our lives. Whether you have been doing this as a parent, an aunty, a teacher, or a friend, we are now watching the children in our lives growing into adults, thriving in their own right, working, educating themselves, and having life experiences of their own—including having children of their own.

We are deep into our careers now, not starting out in the work force and many of us are thinking about what retirement could look like or even fully in it. We are at a place that we are satisfied with the work we have already done, and we are ready to put in the time and energy to focus just a little more on ourselves in a loving and exciting new way.

This includes opening up to creative projects. You may find you have a book to be written and dance to be danced, a quilt to be stitched or Harley to be ridden down the Pacific Coast! Whatever you have still to express is going to start coming to the surface in this next stage in your life, so we are preparing ourselves to act on those creative impulses that arise in us. We are preparing the soil for our growth.

We are not in the stage of life where we are accumulating things. We now see the value of accumulating experiences. You may find you are passing on many of the things you have accumulated. With more time behind us than ahead, we start to be choosy about our experiences, too, only giving our precious, non-renewable time to people, places and things we truly value. Putting our time and efforts into the people, places and things that value us also! When we apply the Pareto Principle, or the 80/20 rule, we may discover that our most valuable relationships reside in

20% of people in our lives. And the remaining 80%? Well, they are more arms-length support staff. Some even begin to fall away as you redirect your time and focus to living your own authentic life.

Reconciling with our present past

It is time to face the very exciting prospect that we are simply not needed in the same ways we have been and that means reclaiming time and energies to thrive in our own lives.

We have outgrown the old or current model and are being brushed by the veil of a more self-inspired way of living. We can see what is on the other side as we look ahead at the footsteps of the women who have walked this road before us. We can most certainly take the leap from our past into our vibrant, present place of re-branding ourselves as we claim the best life ever for ourselves in as many different ways as there are fiery and fabulous women who are getting up close and personal with themselves and each other holding ourselves accountable to lean in and live!

I extend my hand to you to take and walk with me into the mystery as we shift our consciousness and step up as leaders, mentors and pioneering souls for all women ready and willing to thrive in the third act of life.

May our commitment to living illuminated by the Eight Sacred Responsibilities be a historical shift for the women in your families, surrounding communities and your ancestral linage, inspired by you and your pioneering soul. May we continue to find creative new ways to honour, respect and enjoy who we are and our many gifts.

Dearest sister, you are an amazing woman setting a stellar example of living a life of authentic happiness supported by a foundation of Sacred Responsibility. It is my great joy to stand beside you, because together we are stronger.

As I offer myself up as your guide through this powerful process of shift, I also ask of you to hold me accountable to the process, too. Let's keep a dialogue flowing and wish the best for each other as together we become the greatest expression of ourselves. United in the process of living from our wildest dreams from our wild, creative hearts we embrace the Sacred Responsibilities as we would embrace a winning lottery ticket. Because when we begin to live from our sweet wild hearts we have most certainly hit the jackpot!

How we hold each other accountable. Read this out loud, often.

When a Sacred Woman holds another accountable she does so with ease and grace, with humour and love. A Sacred Woman will always see our beauty even on the days we can't see it ourselves. When a Sacred Woman holds us accountable we feel respected and inspired by her and we learn from the Sacred Woman how to hold our own selves accountable in Sacred Responsibility without judgment or shame.

Rebranding at Corporate Headquarters

A rebranding at corporate headquarters is what we are looking at here. In the same spirit of rebranding a company with a new logo, new stylish uniforms, enhancing a great product and a fresh hook line to draw a new kind of customer closer, we, too, embark on a protocol to rebrand ourselves and our attitude towards living out the next stage of our life.

Using the idea of rebranding ourselves much like a company would do is a fun and inspiring way to look at the shifts we are about to make and how we take responsibility for creating a new experience in our lives. The Eight Sacred Responsibilities offer simple practices and the steps we take to launch our new brand. A rebranded and truly authentic self that is ready, resilient and resourceful.

This is a movement of women over fifty taking full responsibility for our happiness and I am asking you to join me. To stand beside me, to hold me accountable to what I am asking of you. It is a book about our sacred responsibility to keep reasonable balance in our lives and to be actively thriving in our gifts. It is a book where I am willing to be vulnerable with you as I try my damndest to Rise the F#ck Up! Sisters, we are in our creative prime and our time is now. And I have no idea why I have taken up swearing lately but I have been enjoying the exclamation point it seems to put on things joining the ranks of the many fabulous women who do what makes them happy and allowing my true authentic swearing-self feel safe to contribute her word-smithing sass! I welcome all parts of me to the table here, the more of me I show up with, the more we can relate to each other.

Over the years I have been blessed to stand beside and help many women who could not seem to give themselves the permission to see past the complicated parts of their lives. To take a few moments to reach out and grab a good laugh or even a few moments to completely relax into full-bodied gratitude. To truly move from our wounds to wisdom together.

Now through this book and The Eight Sacred Responsibilities we expand our community of women who stand beside each other, who help keep each other's hearts held safe and who mentor each other along the way as we learn to love our lives from this new perspective of fiery and fabulous women over fifty!

Together we are entering into an exciting movement of change, sustainable change. A movement of women advocating for happiness. Happiness for themselves and each other. What the world needs now is more people who are willing to quit the cycle of complaining, disappointment and gossip and step into a new way of being in life. Now is the best time ever to shift from our wounds to our wisdom and be the leaders, mentors, and change makers we naturally are simply by reclaiming our own vibrancy through Sacred Responsibility.

Sustainable change makes for thriving people and introducing gentle shifts, creating positive new ways to view life in a simple and steady way will be our way of maintaining our enthusiasm for the practices. We are re-establishing our enthusiasm for taking responsibility for our own happiness and by doing that, the happiness of those closest to us. Because happiness is contagious, we are in the position of writing the guide book! We are women in our third act and are at the head of the table. We are indeed the matriarchs of the third act and we can create a life that rises and shines so brightly that we are the beacons of light humanity is calling for. It is our time to shine!

If we demand of ourselves that we *immediately* become our thriving vibrant self as soon as we have read the last page in this book, we will not have built a strong sustainable foundation. We are going for change that we can sustain, and this change takes the desire to live your most authentic life, a commitment to doing things that are most true to who you are. (the things that increase your energy) It takes patience, and effort. It takes an empowered gentleness and it takes igniting our inner passion and joy for the sacredness of human responsibility. Let us lead ourselves easefully with our light, with our fire, with our illuminated hearts.

I am committed to you. I commit to being one of your greatest cheerleaders. I believe in you and I am grateful for every thread in the tapestry that makes up the divine, unique warrior of a woman you are. I believe in us...May our path be blessed.

FOUNDATIONS

Our Thoughts, Words and Actions

Our thoughts, words, and actions are the foundations of how we communicate who we are at in any given moment and situation. They are the ingredients that make up our personality. So, the quality of our thoughts, words, and actions will be directly related to the quality of our lives. Period. And at this stage of the game, we are our own quality control board. We choose how we think, what we say, and how we move in this life.

Your personality creates your personal reality.
—Dr. Joe Dispenza

We get to choose how we express ourselves in our lives and moving into this third act, this extra adult life, we have the opportunity and capability to consciously create our reality.

Taking Sacred Responsibility for the quality of our thoughts

It is time to lovingly call, "timeout". When we find ourselves consciously creating an elaborate backstory to fight for our disappointment, to stand vigilant for all that has hurt us even if it was decades ago we have got to call ourselves out and take responsibility for the current opportunity of happiness that we have access to right now.

We need to shine a light on the limiting beliefs that have held us back from enjoying our lives and living from the most authentic places within ourselves. While we re-establish and cultivate the things that increase our vitality as our own more natural system of beliefs, we mourn our losses, grieve our life's pains and deeply feel our experiences as part of the process of tending to our hearts. W honour everything about our past, honouring all the terrains we have walked on our journey, honouring each thread of the tapestry that makes up the life we have lived. We stand in our powerful wisdom of each experience.

Our past experiences are part of the foundation that make us strong enough to stand beside another in pain, our past pain is also our building blocks of radical resilience. Our past pain, disappointments and wounds are our battle scars, they do not define us, instead they are proof of our resilience and a powerful reminder of our strength. May we gracefully stand as a shining example of women resilient, battle scars our proof that every day we rise again.

We stand here, now, ready to rewire our brain for radical resilience through self-care, rising and shining, knowing ourselves, collaborating with one and other, creating and playing, relaxing and celebrating and being grateful for the opportunity to do it.

Thoughts—Our imagination practices

Our imagination practice has the power to put us right in the center of change, shifts and new ways of thinking about ourselves and our life well lived. We begin today with using our creative genius to take our thoughts to any and all places imaginable.

We have a plan, and the very action of planning a well-lived life in our imagination practice is our way of installing new circuits in our brain that look like the experience has already happened. You read that right. Imagining our plan or our journey fires up the circuitry, creating new pathways in the brain.

Do not dwell on what you don't want.
—Dalai Lama

And our imagination will lead us directly into feeling when we focus completely on our imagery. The mind does not know the difference between something going on in our outer environment or our inner environment, but it will draw towards us what we think/imagine/meditate or ponder.

We use our imagination practice to create a greater state than we currently feel, and this applies even when we feel fabulous. We use our imagination practice to continually expand our creative plan for ourselves and all we do to kick off the plan is to begin to imagine it in all of its glitter and glory. There are no limits to our imagination. Leave no new idea unexplored.

Dr. Joe Dispenza teaches us about how we use our thoughts and says:

"If you can't think greater then you feel right now, then you are thinking in the past." I loved the first time I heard him say that! This is a life truth we have not been taught in school.

And here is some more interesting information. We think sixty to seventy thousand thoughts per day. Ninety percent of those are the same thoughts as the day before. The brain is an amazing thing, we set up pathways through our growth experiences in life and they get locked in

The true sign of intelligence is not knowledge but imagination.

—Albert Einstein

and as we live our lives the brain is constantly delivering us data to keep us organized and in a place of relying on the data we have created from our experiences. We don't wake up each day and have to relearn how to brush our teeth or put our shoes on, the data has been stored and available for reference it is our fabulous personal data bank. Lucky for us whomever said, "you can't teach an old dog new tricks" has been proven wrong.

In a great article by Debbie Hampton she makes it simple to understand, "…neuroplasticity is an umbrella term referring to the ability of your brain to reorganize itself, both physically and functionally, throughout your life due to your environment, behaviour, thinking, and emotions."

Our environment is a key player and we will come back to that later (the link to her full article is in the reference section at the back).

Scientific research tells us that our brain grows. The brain is malleable. This knowledge has been understood for the last century but now advances in technology can show it to us through brain scan imaging.

We know our brains grow and reorganize themselves, so what I'm interested in, ladies, is getting deeper into that ten percent of our daily thoughts that are not a repeat of the day before. I am interested in all of the space and opportunity to grow our brains, increase our creative thoughts and build new pathways in the brain so that when it is doing its day to day work of keeping us tapped into our data storage it is continually being replenished and updated with plenty of great new material to reference and begin living from.

In his very interesting book, *The Brain That Changes Itself*, Norman Doidge describes the brain "more like a living creature with an appetite, one that can grow and change itself with proper nourishment and exercise."

Our conscious thoughts and our environment create our reality, so back to Dr. Joe. If we are thinking in the past we are functioning from that ninety percent of repeated thought data and normally that is awesome, but there is scientific evidence showing us that time and time again when people change their thoughts and focus on something greater than they currently feel, the entire body responds in ways that decrease stress.

Drop the mic.

What I am suggesting here is that us fiery and fabulous women over fifty are going to make our practices our key to growing our

You have to act as if it were possible to radically transform the world. And you have to do it all the time.

—Angela Davis.

brains, living as resilient beings in our bodies, and reducing the stress in our lives so that we may model a life well-lived to future generations.

Words—Our breathing exercises
Of all the exercises, our breathing exercises are the ones that continue to surprise me with their effectiveness and power and by how much my students and I benefit from them, every time.

We are co-creators in this on both an individual level and a collective level. We are tapping into and unleashing our own personal creative force which in turn aligns us with the greater creative force that we are all breathing from and animated by.

When you do your practices, stand firm in the knowledge that your breath work, body work, and work of your imagination are your new superpowers because we are shifting, changing and re-writing our script from our old story to our new story. What we are doing through this practice can very well be the new normal for the generations to follow. Where it is not only normal to have a "love your life" attitude, but it is encouraged, modelled and encoded into the field.

You may come to this point in your life with your own breathing practices and knowledge of the breath as an ally and anchor. I encourage you to apply your practices in harmony with the breathing practices I put forward here. Be creative, adapt the breathing practices you already have in place and enjoy the ride.

For those who are new to having a breathing practice or a focus on breathing to reduce stress, focus the mind and cleanse the body, welcome! You are going to *love* putting yourself right into the flow of this life-force enhancing practice the yogis call *pranayama*, which loosely translates into life-force regulation or lengthening.

A focused breathing practice supports us in lengthening our lives, because if we are not breathing we are not living, and if we are not breathing well, we are not living well. What we do in our practice is to begin to observe the quality of our breathing from a place of understanding the full potential of this part of our practice. Our breathing exercises balance, energize and recharge our vital energy.

The quality of both our breath and our thoughts determine our state of mind. There is a reason that when someone is really upset we direct them to breathe, to take a deep breath and tell us what is wrong. We all know this medicine. We all know that a few deep breaths before any activity that needs our full attention will focus us. We know that a few deep breaths when we realize we have been holding our breath brings a whole new sensation of ease into our mind and bodies.

We are going for mastery in this area, ladies. Our breath is our anchor in life, and our go-to practice the moment we find ourselves in stress, in fear and in rumination over things we cannot control. The moment your mind starts to have thoughts of uncertainty, that you don't know what to do, what decision to make or where to turn, make it your priority to focus on your breathing. This will bring you to a clearer minded and grounded place from which to make your choices, including the choice to be patient with yourself. Understanding the power within your breath will be a game changer.

We have the ability to reconcile lost or leaked energy through our breathing exercises, we can reduce stress and tension in the body and mind, and we can change the quality and the level of our own energy by being fully committed to a conscious breathing practice. This is radical Sacred Responsibility! For our breathing exercises, we always breathe in through the nose and out through the nose unless instructed otherwise. If you feel light headed during our practices simply take breaks, pause and continue when it feels right for you. We have plenty of time together, there is no need to rush any of our practices, especially our breathing.

If you consider that our breathing is happening whether we focus on it or not, then we owe our breath a lot of gratitude! We go about our day-to-day routines and hardly think about the breath and the life-force that is animating us, yet we are in a continued state of deep relationship with our breath. Perhaps if anything, it is time to honour the people, places and things we are in deep relationship with through our renewed respect for our breath. We are in the flow of our life guided by our breath, slowing down, taking life in fully, and allowing ourselves to be soothed by our breath like the flow of ocean waves moving in and out. Air is free, so fill up your energetic bank account and make conscious breathing practices a priority and your Sacred Responsibility.

All hail the exhale!
Your exhale is your power play. For me it has been a life saver. Counterintuitive, as it would make more sense that

the inhale would really be the defining moment of life or death, but I discovered the power of the exhale and its ability to shift me back into my power at a time of my own depleted energy.

On the exhale our diaphragm is activated in a way that pushes up and it includes muscles of our abdomen in its execution. You activate a power place in your body on the exhale. Notice it now, on your next exhale squeeze out all the air. The area of your body you are feeling now is the place I am bringing to your attention.

In yogic philosophy we talk about this place in the body as an energy center, an energy organ called a chakra. It is called *Manipura*, meaning "lustrous gem." It is the third chakra and it resides in the solar plexus area of our body. It is from this place we relate to the consciousness of our personal power, our willpower and our self-esteem. It is from this place I regained my own strength and reclaimed my depleted energy and got back to living my empowered life and this is why I say, "All hail the exhale"!

In the yogic traditions, we learn that our body has seven main energy centers where we can focus on an alignment that maintains our vitality. The seven main energy centres (chakras/Wheel) are found from the base of our spine to the crown of our head. Our movement, meditation and breathing practices are all sources of tending to our energy body and the balance of our vital life force. Our practices assist us in keeping the energy system in our body flowing, and clear of blockages. It's not unlike a log jam in a river. For various reasons through our life experiences, our environment, the quality of our thoughts and how we care for ourselves these energy centres can become blocked and over time cause us dis-ease in the body. For a crash course in chakras, see Appendix I.

Begin to make your exhale as much of a superstar as your inhale, your exhale holds its own powerful force that we now elevate and bring into its rightful position of honour in our lives.

Oh, and I highly encourage inhaling also, they make a great team. It is helpful to have at least a beginner's knowing that these energetic organs exist as everything we are doing together rides on maintaining our fiery and fabulous vital life force.

Learn how to exhale, and the inhale will take care of itself.
—Carla Melucci Ardito

Actions—Our physical exercises
The physical part of the practice is built on an understanding that there is something for everyone. As we change from day to day, getting physically stronger or occasionally being challenged in our bodies, we will always have a movement practice we are able to participate in. On the days you have high energy increase your time and effort on the physical practice. On the days you have lower energy chose the more simplified variations.

Our movement practice will keep us in a consistent flow of caring for our bodies. It will maintain a "tuned in" state of our energy levels, our strength, flexibility and our coordination day to day, and we can adjust our movement accordingly. If we are not tuned into our physical body each day we may indeed miss something of substance, something that we would want to tend to. If we notice that we are losing flexibility or strength in an area, we can bring more focus and care to that area.

These are simple rules of self-care: move your body, pay attention to your body's needs and tend to them. Our physical practice deepens and for many of us will awaken a new connection to our body. Loving our awesome over-fifty body is a Sacred Responsibility. It is the vessel for our beautiful hearts.

In a world full of busying ourselves, moving here and moving there, filling up our schedules and an underlying fear of missing out (FOMO) there is movement. There is physical action and movement in all this rushing around that we understand and relate to as satisfying in some way. The old program we have been running, where we base our self-worth on the length of our to-do list, is obsolete. That kind of movement is *not* the same as consciously caring for our bodies with a physical movement practice.

It is that movement we approach with reverence, like a prayer. We all have an understanding that moving our bodies is indeed beneficial. We have less of an understanding (or interest at times) that tending to our thoughts/mind or our breathing as an exercise is equally important. So, for our fast-paced culture we typically meet at the physical first. Then, as if by some magical understanding our yoga teacher bestows on us about the breath and the mind while we are in a physical activity (my bestie likes to say 'to socialize the idea') we begin to find the mind and breath exercises more interesting. But inevitably we will all meet in agreement that moving our body is important especially as we grow wiser. Use it or lose it, right!

We will continue to create audios and videos of our practices making them available to support and enjoy the movements together, and just because they seem easy do not discount their potential to keep you strong, flexible and totally tuned into your body. (Links to our videos are on www.reachyogalifestyle.ca Just enter the Sacred Portal to access them.)

We are embarking on our life as a moving meditation and our practices are designed to slow us down a little, to get to know ourselves more deeply and in that experience a deepened relationship with ourselves.

One of the things that is genius about getting into a 'moving meditation' rhythm with our bodies is that it is a stable bridge from our previous lives that had us moving extremely fast, into this new smooth, sultry way of enjoying life in our bodies. I'm finding myself luxuriating in life more, taking the day-to-day things a little slower, the sound track from *Burlesque* playing in my head... I am definitely more in my body than ever before. This is part of the power of a woman in her third act!

It has been a process getting to this place of ease in my body. I didn't expect myself to stop on a dime the day I turned fifty and overnight emerge from the chrysalis a graceful, sultry butterfly. Quite the opposite. I had plans! But as those years have passed now and I have gained a clearer picture of how genius the physical practices have been for me during the transition into my fifty's I will shout it from the mountain tops.

Keep moving your beautiful body!

As we transition into our third act together, taking Sacred Responsibility for ourselves, we enjoy our movement, maintain our energy and we can put the brakes on as fast or as slowly as we like. You don't see the Grandmothers rushing around the fire at a Ceremony now do you? Watch them. They are the physical embodiment of cool and calm. (I love you Grandmother Vera, thank you for teaching how me kick-ass gentleness is!)

As in any of our practices we work up slowly no matter how "easy" you think the exercises are. We are cultivating focus on a whole new level now. We are way too fabulous to rush our practices. Our minds are cool and calm, and we are building our resilience one breath at a time.

Have no doubt there is plenty of time and room for joining a running group or to take up hiking or any number of physical activities but for now we practice simple movements for strength, flexibility, balance, cleansing and overall connection to our beautiful bodies.

Feeling it

It seems that every section of the book I write is the most important part of the book. Because it all matters, the tapestry of all of the sections of the book making up the wholeness of the message of our movement. But I'm going to point out that feeling our positive emotions, shifting into a moment of truly feeling our happiness, our joy, our enthusiasm, or any number of positive emotions to assist us to move forward in a fabulous state of well-being may indeed be the most important part of our work together. Keep this idea in your mind until it makes its way into your heart and into your body. We are aligning our thoughts and feelings with our plan of a life well lived. Feeling it is where it's at.

Feelings move through us on a stream of chemical reactions cascading through our bodies. We will have streams of "happy" chemicals—dopamine, serotonin, oxytocin and endorphin—and we are also up against "stress" hormones, cortisol, noradrenaline, adrenaline. Obviously, we will feel fabulous when bathed in happy chemicals and not so fabulous when bathed in stress hormones. But before we go throwing the baby out with the bath water, we want all our chemicals available and working for us. We are taking Sacred Responsibility for our happiness and will have our focus on creating positive experiences in our lives by making a conscious choice, as a practice, to intentionally play with positive more balanced responses to life. We are working with our brains ability to create new pathways, new ways of seeing ourselves and our place in this world. *And* we don't disrespect our stress chemicals in the process. Our brain is so incredibly tuned in that we will be in a dance of chemical reactions that are all doing their best to keep us safe and alive, and we will need to learn how best to take the lead.

Conversations on happiness are no longer left up to the philosophers and artists, scientists now have a huge impact on what we know about feelings and happiness. So, as we take a deepened interest in our happiness we can find our paths through the arts, the sciences and the philosophical discussions that support our journey of reclaiming happiness as a respected attribute in life. Rise and Shine!

The Laws of Attraction
There are many folks having this discussion about attracting things into our lives and the best ways to do it. I have a couple of things to say about this. As we embark on a revised way of living our lives in this second maturity we begin to take note of what contributes to our energy reserves and what depletes our energy reserves. It will take time and effort to sort out one from the other, the people, places and things that lift us up or bring us down. But as we slowly wade through these conversations the one thing we can be sure of is whatever we put our focus on we will magnetize towards us. We will attract to us the things we focus on.

In order to "attract" the very best for us it only makes sense to focus on the very best things, right? Technically yes, but we are in a place of change in our lives and while we are making shifts and changes it is important that we are patient with ourselves. Some days we will not waiver on our gratitude for this life and some days we will wonder what the heck we are doing here. Remember even in the plan to attract to us the people, places and things that light us up we will have many moments of discouragement and wishing for a quicker leap into our fabulous third act.

If you truly understand that our thoughts words and actions will attract to us what we are thinking, saying, and doing we will be able to have the deeper conversations with ourselves about exactly what it is we desire to attract or magnetize. We will learn how to upgrade our ways of thinking about ourselves and our environment so that we experience what we desire in the present moment.

Now normally I am a big supporter of the statement, "you are never too old to…" fill in your own blank. But there is one exception to that rule and that is, "we are *way* to old not to enjoy our lives".

So, let's get on with it as my Grandmother Marguerite would say!

Chapter One

THE FIRST SACRED RESPONSIBILITY: SELF-CARE

Good health is not just an absence of symptoms; it's the presence of high energy, endless stamina, creative intelligence, an interest in work, and a peaceable disposition.
                                                            —Penny Kelly

I know, who has time for self-care these days right? We have filled our lives to the brim, and if that is not enough we cruise the real estate sites and vacation sites looking for the next big trip, that dream home, that thing to run to or distract us from being present to our own self-care responsibilities. The first item on the agenda is to dissolve the illusion of Self-Care as Selfishness.

Dissolving the Illusion of Self-Care as Selfishness
Self-care will look vastly different for all of us.

Self-Care is the First Sacred Responsibility and it is the most difficult one to fully embrace, especially for women. It is the one Sacred Responsibility that will push our buttons and the buttons of those closest to us. We need to reprogram our mindset to include moments throughout our day where we fully acknowledge and embrace doing something good for us without judgment.

When we prioritize self-love, our Self-Care practices are done with reverence and we are inspired to love and care for ourselves. This means we do not need to make up an excuse to do the things that increase our vitality.

It means being true to the activities that lift us up and being truthful with ourselves around the activities that deplete us. Sometimes that will mean saying no to invitations that decrease our energy and yes to staying in with our feet up reading a great book. Or, saying no thanks to an evening of sitting around rehashing the same old dusty conversations and instead going out dancing.

The simple self-care protocol directs us to fully experience the self-care we are giving ourselves. This means that when we pause for three sweet deep breaths we no longer push through them like a task. Oh no, sisters, we luxuriate in those three breaths, we breathe sensuality into our cells as we breathe with our full presence to our own self-care.

Interestingly enough, when we do things that are good for *us* everyone benefits. Our families and communities benefit more from us when we come from a place where we are grounded in a solid foundation of self-respect, self-care and self-awareness. Everyone wins when we treat ourselves well and with loving-kindness. When we make our self-development an exciting activity it gives everyone around us permission to do the same, and it becomes contagious.

Having practices that support self-care, respect and love for life, and a commitment to taking responsibility for our happiness builds a solid foundation for getting our balance back when we are hit with the unexpected. It also establishes an understanding of the importance of inner peace. I know that when the shit hits the fan we are not feeling so Zen. That's ok, dive in and feel it all fully. It is your shit hitting the fan, take responsibility for it, learn from it and grow in the process.

We now take Sacred Responsibility for our Self-Care by pioneering a new way of living. Living in an empowered mindset without believing the old programs like "if someone catches us caring for ourselves, that means we are not working hard enough". As we get honest with ourselves and embrace the things that increase our vitality, the old programs can begin to dissolve, but not until we truly understand that we are worthy of choosing self-care. In order to thrive in the First Sacred Responsibility of Self-Care we must end the belief that we need to give excuses for our choices to do the things that increase our energy and make us happy. No-one said we had to say yes to every great invitation we receive. Say no and use that time for Self-Care and your self-development.

Anyone who has flown on a commercial airplane knows that the safety rules tell us to put on our own oxygen mask then put our child's mask on. This is direct and to the point, the rules tell us to look after ourselves first and others second. Mentally, I get it. Make sure we are strong and capable so that we are able to look after the more vulnerable in our lives. Emotionally, I'm not so sure about choosing myself over the child or Elder beside me. But what I *can* relate to, is this as a metaphor for day-to-day life. That if I commit to self-care now and maintain a certain level of health in my mind and body that if the time comes when I am in one of these situations I will be prepared and able to respond swiftly from a place of strength and clarity. Because I have been wearing my own oxygen mask all along.

Take three luxurious breaths and hold space for yourself to receive that it is ok to put yourself first right now.

Inhale, retain, exhale, pause....
Inhale, retain, exhale, pause....
Inhale, retain, exhale, pause....

What would it take to get inspired enough to put your self-care in a position of high priority in your daily life? To become personally inspired, to truly know Self-Care as a Sacred Responsibility. Does the Universe really need to take you out with a health issue or an injury for you to know that you are worthy of all the care you give out to others?

I hear it time and time again, women telling me how they were forced into self-care because of sickness or injury and this takes a little piece of my heart each time I hear their stories. What I do know is that things happen, we get sick and hurt whether it be heart, mind, or body, things happen. I also know that how we live our lives has a direct impact on how quickly or slowly we heal and bounce back from illness, injury and disappointment.

Living Large
As a thriving woman over fifty, I am not about to allow myself to miss out on the fullness of life and the fullness of

life will, at times, include what it feels like to lose someone, to feel hurt in a situation and to feel a broken heart.

I am up for a rich life and all experiences, all emotions and all responses that are available to me and I am committed to being fully responsible to the ways I respond to the tough stuff in my life. Over my life I have learned that reacting is never as good for me as responding. I have also learned that it is a gift of self-love to allow myself to be honest, authentic and vulnerable and to stand up for those parts of myself. I have learned not to dim my light and my love of life even when I have been sucker-punched (metaphorically) by those I held closest to me.

I have learned that I am indeed resilient and that I will not do a disservice to the hard things in life by allowing myself to be happy. The truth is that happiness and upset can live just fine together. I do not need to cut happiness out of my life because I am experiencing something challenging, both can live harmoniously together. The trick is hitting the sweet spot where we allow for the experience without being all-consumed. Balance is found in that sweet spot, just like in a yoga posture.

I will be honest, my preference is a life of rainbows, butterflies and dancing my ass off to loud music but I know that it is *all* of my life experiences, great and not so great that make me unique. It enables me to be an example for someone else to see that we are incredible, resilient and wonderful humans who get back up no matter how hard we have been knocked down. But in the end, the quality of our life and our experiences will depend on where we choose to focus our attention—on the pain or the joy.

The Story of the Two Wolves

This is a beautiful traditional story, passed down in slightly different variations but it is a story that continues to inspire me, so I share it here. With gratitude to the Indigenous Story Tellers of Turtle Island, if not for you I may have forgotten everything.

One evening a Cherokee Elder told his grandson about a battle that goes on inside people. He said, "My son, the battle is between two wolves inside us all. It is a terrible fight between these two wolves. One is evil—he is anger, envy, sorrow, regret, greed, arrogance, self-pity, guilt, resentment, inferiority, lies, false pride, superiority, and ego."

He continued, "The other is good—he is joy, peace, love, hope, serenity, humility, kindness, benevolence, empathy, generosity, truth, compassion, and faith. The same fight is going on inside you—and inside every other person, too."

The grandson thought about it for a minute and then asked his grandfather, "Which wolf will win?"

The Cherokee Elder simply replied, "The one you feed."

Self-Care and having a plan

When you are in a place in your life where you feel you have not found a way to cope it can be difficult to stay focused on self-care. We have all been there for one reason or another, many times. Yet here we are today creating our plan for living joyously with our past stresses behind us and in many cases forgotten completely.

We now have our practices and refreshed mindset and taking sacred responsibility for our happiness every day is our bold move to build up our resilience and our coping skills.

We have a plan to thrive

Do not forget we have a plan. When we take responsibility for our emotional health as well as our physical and mental health we are hitting the holy trinity of living like our authentic human selves. I cannot stress this point enough— the simplicity of our practices is actually the path.

Even though all of us fiery and fabulous women over fifty are embarking on many creative projects that may feel like we are starting a new career with all the bells and whistles and late nights that our projects can take, *this* time around, we come at our second adult life from a place of simplicity. This new time in our life is indeed rich with activity, yet now we have released our need to attach stress to our activities. Now, we find ourselves actively creating without the stress program playing. This is one of the benefits of being over fifty!

We are fiery, fabulous and at peace with who we are. If you are not there yet, we have your back and we are getting there together. Our self-care practices include making choices for ourselves that are authentic for us at this time in our lives.

Go grey, burn your bra, get streaks, eat salads, drink bourbon, dance all night long, nap in the sunshine. Just be you. It is your time to be authentically you.

Self-Care as a Sacred Responsibility has just as much to do with the care of our body as it does with the care of our heart and mind. We tend to our self-care in a holistic way where we look at our whole life including the environment we live in. Be ready, resilient and resourceful when it comes to Self-Care. Know what things bring you more energy and what things deplete your energy. This is a big part of where to begin for all of us, when immersed in Sacred Self-Care we find ourselves more often in the places that feel the best, with the people who treat us the best, doing the things that we love best. Every day we preform tiny devotional rituals, slowly restoring self-honour that in turn make powerful shifts in our lifestyle and personal attitude.

By choosing a new way of treating ourselves we ignite a new way of responding in our lives that is more authentic, more easeful, and more fun!

Our Self-Care and the needs of others

Part of being fiery and fabulous over fifty is that we are imbued with the gift of being capable of personal Self-Care *and* still having our antenna up for anyone we care about who needs us to care for them. We have many years under our belt of caring for other people, so it is easy to shift that kind of focus onto ourselves now, and still be available to shift our care expertise to someone close to us whenever they may be in need.

Even though we are enjoying putting the focus on us in this changing time in our lives, caring for others is like riding a bike for us and we don't have to forget others to tend to our own self-care. We can do both, because our practices are simple, powerful and takes just a few minutes a day. We have plenty of time for the days someone else is in need *and* we will be more grounded and helpful then we have been in the past when we are called upon.

"But I don't have time for self-care."
I hear this often and I have even thought it. Then one day I hit the jackpot! A depth of understanding flooded over me, and I knew in my bones that when I get up and wash my face and brush my teeth I have immersed myself in Self-Care as a Sacred Responsibility.

I began to pay attention to this morning ritual, to treat it as a prayer of gratitude to start my day. I began to *feel* the moment of gratitude and appreciation for the day, for the fresh water and for my healthy teeth and my shiny eyes in the mirror. I began to be fully present to what I was doing each morning and that indeed I had been acting in Self-Care as a Sacred Responsibility all along! I realized that I could no longer honestly say, "I didn't make time for any self-care today", that I was fully immersed in it upon awakening.

This was a game changer for me. So, sisters, this is where it begins.

Today you start by honouring what you already do. I know you have a self-care practice already and I am happily going to expose you right now. Yes you, who gets up each morning and takes a few deep breaths and stretches even before you put your feet on the floor. When it is done with intent and mindfulness you have a morning yoga ritual in place already! You cat-stretch yourself in to the day, drawing in deeply on your inhale. This indeed is the way to start a day in self-care.

Or, you take a few minutes to journal your dreams and creative ideas in those first moments of wakefulness. You have a practice of self-care for your creativity! For those of us with creaking bodies and whose deep breaths are more moans as we hit the snooze button, you are not out of the spot light of my exposing your current self-care practice either. Stumbling to the bathroom, you wash your face and brush your teeth preparing to present yourself to the day. You have a self-care practice.

If you are reading this book it is likely that you are blessed with clean water and a toothbrush. Start looking at that as a blessing and brushing your teeth as a self-care ritual.

We begin the road to re-establishing our connection to Self-Care by honoring what we are doing right now, and I mean truly honouring it.

From this moment forward each time you brush your teeth and wash your hands I'd like you to get into it like it is the best thing you could ever do for yourself. Stay present to the few moments it takes to perform the self-care ritual of brushing your teeth. Get to know the inside of your mouth, each tooth and your tongue. Get to know what is going on in there! This is the place that all your beautiful words flow from. It's the place you speak your truth from, the place you taste nourishment from and most importantly this is the place you laugh from. Begin now to give it the honour and respect it deserves.

Visionary Barbra Marx Hubbard tells us, "your voice carries the great creative process in you". With this in mind, tend to your brushing as if you are establishing your own artist's palate. From here your most creative songs and stories can emerge and inspire.

The S Word

Stress. The World Health Organization has called stress the Global Health epidemic of the 21st century. Stress and the amount of energy we give to stressful situations in our lives will be a very important place to observe our responses.

It's true. Life can be messy at times and some days it will be more difficult than others to find our center. It requires approaching our stress in a way that allows for every possible stress-reduction tool to be considered. We don't have to be a victim of our stress. In some cases, a little stress can light our fire and get us moving and shaking things up. While we practice the techniques of stress management, we are taking Sacred Responsibility for our stress reduction through the Eight Sacred Responsibilities.

Let me remind you what they are so that you may read them slowly and let then sink into your awareness. Self-Care, Rise and Shine, Know Yourself, Collaborate, Honour your Intuition, Create and Play, Relax and Celebrate and Gratitude are all paths to a life where you are not operating from a place of high stress when it is not appropriate to be stressed. Remember we are building our resilience so that we become better able to re-establish balance for ourselves during challenge and change and the demands of life.

Stress is not only an issue when big life problems arise. It is the accumulated stress that sneaks up on us and can make us sick. Two excellent websites for those of you who would like to get a deeper understanding of how stress effects our lives, or the lives of those we care for, are both in the resource section at the back of the book. I highly recommend reading the website materials posted on both *The Alignment Project* and *Heart Math*.

A sample from the Alignment Project's web site:

> Research shows that even one stressful situation pro-
> motes a cascade of over 1,400 biochemical changes in
> the body, producing harmful hormones like Cortisol
> and depleting our bodies of regenerative hormones,
> like DHEA, also known as the vitality hormone.

Pick your battles
Understanding this can be a very successful way to come
back to center when overwhelmed with stress. We simply
do not need to take on everything for everyone in every
moment…we just don't. Find out what amount of your
stress is self-inflicted and begin to gently undo yourself
from overwhelm. One item at a time, one breath at a time.
Do not let anyone rush you. Take full responsibility for any
stress that you have chosen. We waste a lot of time blaming
others when we have so much unnecessary stress we could
liberate ourselves from. Breathe, realize, respond if even
just with yourself.

Respond
Let your thoughts, words and actions be a response not
a reaction. As we establish practices of stress reducing activities we begin to respond with deeper understanding of
any situation where we are stressed. Reducing our levels of
stress is a practice. In some situations, we are able to be the
one who keeps calm and carries on, other days we are sure
it's the worst day ever. Somewhere on the middle path lies
the practice. Begin to pay attention to what the signals of
stress are for you.

Heart Centered Listening

Sometimes the strength of a sacred woman can be mistaken for her not having problems, pains or heartaches. It is easy to not hear her when a strong woman is trying to say she is not coping, because she has been strong her whole life. As women of wisdom we cultivate our deep listening skills. We go inward and listen intently to our own inner voice. It is our responsibility to hear our own calling and our wise inner guidance for ourselves so that indeed we thrive. As we cultivate these listening skills by practicing on ourselves, we develop deeper listening skills for others. This focused listening is also known as Heart Centered listening. Practice being a deep listener, as listening is not passive at all, it is fully active. Did you know that the quality of your heart centered listening can calm the person speaking? We can defuse upset and calm each other when we practice heart centered listening with one another.

Inhale, retain, exhale and pause…Inhale, retain, exhale and pause…

Inhale, retain, exhale and pause… And listen…

(Listen and silent are made up of the exact same letters.)

Become Open to Possibilities

Become more open to the possibility of a stress-free day. We are here to live our lives fully and that includes stress free days, plenty of them! If we are stuck in an old idea that "life is stressful" it will be more difficult to see the shiny stuff going on all around us. Remember Dr. Joe? If we can't think greater then we feel right now, then we are thinking in the past.

Life can be stressful, and it can be peaceful and joyous, loving and downright hilarious. Life can be everything, so become open to other possibilities outside of stress.

Be mindful of your thoughts, words and actions as these are the foundations of how you communicate, these are the foundations of how you show up in the world.

Sleep, The Other S Word

If we don't sleep well all our systems suffer. Most people are in their greatest state of rejuvenation from sleep when they get 7-8 hours per night. This changes with age, younger people need a little more, older people need a little less and each of us has our own sweet spot when it comes to a good night's rest. We all know the difference of how we feel energized and clear minded when we are well rested, just as much as we know how sluggish and discombobulated we feel when we didn't sleep well.

It takes courage to say yes to rest and play in a culture where exhaustion is seen as a status symbol.
—Brené Brown

This is basic stuff, sisters, and it is serious stuff. Our body, mind and spirit all need sleep to thrive. When we sleep we are in a deep state of self-care, all of our organs rest, our mind rests, our body rests. We enter the dream-time state where we can catch glimpses of stories from our own inner spirit world. This is a non-negotiable part of our self-care practice.

In Lesley Stahl's article, *The Science of Sleep,* she writes that world-wide large-scale studies report a link between short deep sleep times and obesity, as well as heart disease, high blood pressure, and stroke. Lack of sleep impacts our appetite, our metabolism, our memory, and how we age. The link to her full article is in the resources section at the back of our book but her conclusion is that when we talk about diet and exercise as our healthy life combination it must include sleep.

I don't want to be downer here but let me conclude the note on sleep with this. Humans are the only ones who treat sleep deprivation is a badge of honour and brag about how much you can accomplish when you don't "waste time" on sleep. We were wrong on that one. Studies prove time and time again, that when we are sleep deprived, when our deep sleep state is interrupted, we get very sick. It is dangerous how deeply our ability to function is compromised. Know yourself, understand the right amount of deep sleep needed for you to be at your best each day. Sleep is a Sacred Responsibility of Self-Care, period.

A few tips on getting a good night's sleep.

Make yourself comfortable. For some of us, it might be time to replace our mattresses, pillows or bedding. Use the resources you have to make the place you sleep as comfortable as possible.

Clear your bedroom of devices. Computers and cell phones in the bedroom? No… just no. In order to fall to sleep in a reasonable amount of time leave your screen time behind when you go to bed. Even better shut off the Wi-Fi when you go to bed. (yeah, that's right, I said it, shut the wi-fi off when you go to bed!)

Soothing Music. If you like to fall asleep with something playing in the background, experiment with music that will lull you to sleep instead of falling asleep to the TV screen. Set a timer so the music drifts off shortly after you do.

Romance. One of the great ways to sleep well and deeply is to fall asleep content with romantic connection. Sex is a great way to reduce tension and anxiety, both of which are big culprits of sleep disturbance. Get romantic, get a good night's sleep.

Before bed bath or shower. Have a warm soak or a brief steamy shower and rinse the busyness of the day down the drain. I call it "the rinse cycle" and it is one of my best sleeping tricks. A five-minute shower clears my mind and relaxes my body for sleep.

Count your blessings. Relax your heart and mind by ending your day with closing your eyes and counting your blessings. Running gratitude through your mind at the end of the day will help to relax you and flood your cells with a feeling of wellbeing.

Romance. Oh, I said that one already… but it is worth repeating.

Water

In my quest to seek out the professionals around me to help me understand how best to serve my body I worked with two of the wisest women in my circle on this and both of them asked me the same two questions first. How much water do you drink a day, and how much sleep are you getting each night?

Remember what we are doing together is taking Sacred

Responsibility for ourselves so that we can move into our third act as a fiery and fabulous woman who is thriving and happy. Make drinking enough water an act of self-care.

I'm being fully transparent with you, sisters, both sleep and water have been a struggle for me. I have had all the excuses in the book to rationalize that I stay up way later than my yoga teacher would ever believe! And I do not drink anywhere near the amount of water that I personally need to feel my best.

I say, "I am a night hawk" or "Oh, I'm not a big drinker", and on and on blah, blah, blah. But when I began to write this book I knew this had to change and it had to change immediately. I was not willing to impart my words of Sacred Responsibility as a sleep-deprived, thirsty gal.

As adult women, we are approximately 55% water (when we were born we were closer to 75% water). It is imperative that we maintain a constant relationship with water as physical coordination and our mental performance become impaired at about 1% dehydration. Water is distributed around our body in a perfect flow. In an article by Dr. Anne Marie Helmenstine PhD, published on *Thought-Co*, September 2018, she answers the question, "Where is water in the human body?"

According to her, two thirds of the body's water is fluid within the cells (intracellular) and one third is extracellular (fluids outside the cells). The heart and brain are 73% water, lungs 83%, muscles and kidneys are 79%, the skin 64%, and the bones are around 31% water.

Dr. Helmenstine goes on to share functions of water in the body: Water is the primary building block of cells. It is used to flush waste from the body and carry oxygen and nutrients to the cells. It acts as an insulator for the brain, spinal cord and organs by acting as a shock absorber. (The link to the full article is in the Resource section at the back of the book).

I believe that when we have more understanding of what our bodies actually require to thrive we will be more likely to make it happen. We don't know until we know and well… now you know. Water is essential to coordination and mental performance, enough said.

> *TIP: Have a personal water jug. Look around at what you already have in your home that could be your fabulous hydration container and fill it up with the best water you have access to and drink up. I find that the majority of people I work with erroneously believe they drink enough water daily. If you have your own jug, you are able to keep a mental note as well as a visual on how much water you are drinking each day. This is an area of my health that matters to me and I have to monitor myself and be sure to drink my jug of water each day! Add drinking your jug of water to your non-negotiable list.*

A Personal Test and The Amazing KG.

The benefits of committing to a more Sacred Relationship with sleep and water were quickly obvious. I did a really big test when I booked myself in a loft cabin in the country for a week to write undisturbed. I also hired one of those fabulous professionals I had been working with to help keep me on track. Working with Nutritionist Kassia Gooding was like hiring a personal trainer for my habits. She prepared meals that were incredibly delicious and fun, she had water drinking requirements of me and she even served me fresh herbs to inhale for cognitive function while writing. The difference in how I felt was amazing, I thought I was feeling fantastic when I got there, then this experiment took everything to the next level. The water and deep sleep were key to how clear minded I felt that week.

I was lucky enough to have a friend and professional in Kassia to help me on this part of the journey. What I needed was to immerse fully into the simplicities of daily health under the guidance of someone who cared about my success as much as I did. It was one of the best things I have ever done for myself. A few weeks back I had a conversation with Kassia and asked her if she would be willing to be our official Holistic Nutritionist. She said, yes! Now our community of fiery and fabulous women has access to her amazing wisdom and loving heart on our journey and she is thrilled to join us!

I have added her web site link to our resources section in the book and we will invite her for online interviews, cooking classes, and she will speak to us on areas that best support women's nutritional health in their third act. Go ahead and write down your questions and we will go to the expert! Welcome to the community, Kassia! (Remember to join our online community through our website so you don't miss any of the fun! www.reachyogalifestyle.ca.)

Simplify Self-Care

Try things, let it be that simple. Just go ahead and try things. Most of us are new to making our self-care a priority and just because we are onto it now doesn't mean every current person and activity gets tossed aside in a frenzy of immediate change.

We will find, more often than not, when we bring into our lives the things that make us feel good, the things that bring us more joy and increase our life force, the things that do not do it for us anymore tend to fall away gently. So, try things out that you intuitively feel would make you happy, contribute to your vitality and that spark your interest.

Get judgment out of your system

You can stop judging yourself right now for what you think are bad habits. Those things will begin to be so out of sync with your new state of being that those habits won't even feel like they belong to you anymore. Go ahead and write down any of the judgements you might be holding around the ways you do the opposite of self-care. Write them down as your first action towards bringing them up and out of your mind and your body.

If you can't think of any ways you judge yourself right now, just know if a self-judgment statement comes to mind later be sure to write it down. Let it come up and out as self-judgment no longer serves your greater good. Now we add a twist, write it in past tense. Remember the subconscious mind doesn't know the difference if we are physically in any given situation or just thinking about a situation, and the subconscious mind will do all that it can to execute our thoughts for us. We are rewiring our thought patterns as we bring the things we judge about ourselves up and out to be transformed.

I used to judge myself for _____

_____

I used to judge myself for_____

_____

I used to judge myself for_____

_____

Walks, baths, tending to your nails and your bodies outermost needs as tiny devotional acts of self-care are simple ways to begin your personal self-care rituals. Begin to pay attention to any areas of your body that are calling out. Your body is highly intelligent, and it will give you signs and signals asking you to take Sacred Responsibility for yourself. A sacred woman pays attention to her body and engages in Self-Care from a state of love for self, respect for her beautiful body, and honour for the life force flowing through her. Self-care body rituals are part of preventive planning. We take care of ourselves as a Sacred Responsibility so that we are not forced into self-care because we chose not to make body care our priority.

Massage as a non-negotiable

One of the best ways you can stay tuned into your body is by self-massage. I put massage in the non-negotiable category because it is self-empowering to have a deep relationship to your physical body. Every inch of your body is waiting for you to love it, to care for it and to enjoy it. We are going for being happy in our physical bodies on this journey. Your muscles work hard for you, treat them with gratitude. Find a nice natural oil that you like. You might like coconut oil, or almond oil. Take a few drops in your hands and begin by massaging your hands and fingers. Take a full minute to do this then sit back feel your body's response to your hands being massaged. Massage your knees, your feet and your forearms, all the places that are easy to reach. Do one area of your body one day, and another area another day if only for a few minutes a couple of times a week. Move from place to place and make your way over every inch of your body eventually starting the process over—well every inch you can reach! We have time and we care about feeling good in our bodies. Make massage a non-negotiable because you love every inch of yourself, inside and out. And, because it feels great!

Each of us will step into our self-care in our own unique way. Many of us may enjoy lots of the same self-care activities, of course, but the way we experience our self-care will be unique to each of us. What we have in common is the willingness and the desire to begin to take Sacred Responsibly for all areas of our lives.

Living in a conscientious way can assist us in deepening our Self-Care practice. We are conscious moving through our daily routine, the way we move from one activity to the next from the way we wake up in the morning to going to bed at end of day. All our daily activities can easily be done consciously. Slow down, observe your surroundings and participate in this life consciously.

Self-Care Tips for the Sacred Woman
- Be true to yourself.
- Give your body the things it loves most.
- Laugh often.
- Sip water all day long.
- Move your body.
- Make massage a non-negotiable.
- Remember that your bones love weight-bearing exercise.
- Enhance the quality of your meals.
- Engage in interesting conversations.
- Enjoy your own company.
- Listen.
- Laugh, dance, make-out, repeat.
- Sleep deeply

Cathy's Self-Care Non-Negotiable
I care for my feet. Start now if you have not yet begun to do this for yourself. You will thank me later if you pick up the non-negotiable Self-Care act of foot care. Thank your feet every day, learn to massage them, moisturize with natural oils, nail care, flexibility and strength. Wear shoes that fit well and are comfortable *and* put your bare feet on the ground. Go for a barefoot walk on the grass. If you are not

comfortable walking barefoot, sit on a chair with your bare feet in the grass. Barefooting is a grounding game changer for us, and we are extremely fortunate to have the Barefoot Pilgrim Sue Kenney in our community.

Her latest book is called, *How to Wear Bare Feet*. I have added it to our reference section. It is full of her experiences of healing her feet, her body and her heart while on the barefoot journey. From Sue's book we learn, "There are no real negative side effects of barefooting. It reverses the aging process, improves brain function, boosts self-esteem and makes you feel happy. It's natural medicine."

And she is so fiery and fabulous that she has even walked El Camino de Santiago barefoot, *many times*! She and I have even done it together. Sue will be showing up to share her wisdom with us online and at our retreats.

Sue and I are exactly one decade apart in age. She is an incredible mentor for me and a shining example of a fiery and fabulous woman in her third act. I always tell her, "I look at you and know pretty much how I will be in ten years."

She is also one of the first women in Canada to be a Certified Wim Hof Method instructor. In case you haven't heard of this yet, Wim Hof is "The Iceman" the amazing man who has taken science by surprise with his three-pillar method of cold plunge (Ice Baths), breathing, and commitment. He continues to break world records and is the subject of extensive research at Stanford University. His purpose is to inspire people to be happy and healthy. We love his plan!

Care for your feet, so you are as comfortable and as mobile as possible always. We have places to go, sisters!

What is your Self-Care Non-Negotiable? Write it down and maintain it and share it to inspire others to choose a self-care non-negotiable. Choose just one self-care non-negotiable and be loyal to it, until it becomes part of who you are. Then choose another one.

My Self-Care Non-Negotiable: _____

_____

Our First Sacred Practice
We Women share in the protocol practices with reverence for the potent possibilities that lie dormant within us. We accept our practice with open hearts and open minds in the knowing that these tiny acts of self-care grow quickly into a renewed love of our lives. We know in every cell of our gorgeous being that our practices fill us with the vibrancy of universal life-force.

Our Daily Statement
Today I open myself fully to living a sacred life, I call in now the people, places and things that lift me up, light me up and hold me up as the accountable, responsible and authentic woman I am here to be. And so it is.

The Self-Care Imagination Practice
(Imagining/Thoughts)

Choose one self-care practice to imagine. It could be any-thing that you feel is key for you to fully embody self-care as a Sacred Responsibility. It can be something you have done in the past or something you dream of doing for yourself one day. It can be as simple as imagining yourself on a beautiful walk in your neighbourhood, or as elaborate as imagining yourself at a private spa in the Swiss Alps. Remember this is your imagination, and nothing is im-possible in your imagination. Once you have chosen the practice, you are going to imagine.

Take a few minutes and close your eyes and begin to see yourself there. Imagine you feel like you are totally com-fortable, you know your way around, and you are rocking this self-care ritual for yourself. Breathe deeply, and relax into your visualization, let your mind wander to all the best places you can take this self-care ritual. Then really begin to feel it, feel like you are there, notice what you are wearing (or not wearing!) notice the atmosphere of your surround-ings. The sounds, the smells, the time of day you are imag-ining. Get into right into it. Take five minutes and go deep into your imagination, practicing feeling your self-care as if you are actually there.

I will share my favorite example to get you going. Some of you may like this one too!

My example: I love to exaggerate my own self-care practices in my mind. It makes me happy and makes me feel like a Goddess!

I love taking long hot baths and I like to feel that I am

soaking in a healing tea. So even though I am in my sweet little apartment in a fifty-year-old 6'x 8' bathroom, in my mind I am in an Egyptian Temple and the high priestess has run my bath. The water is the purest water from deep in the earth. It feels like I am bathing in silk. The fragrance is intoxicating and there are flower petals floating upon bubbles. The tub is made of alabaster and it amplifies the beneficial properties of the healing bath. The steamy, mysterious fragrance of essential oils rises from the water and candlelight flickers dancing shadows on the walls. This is most certainly heaven. I am served tea while I soak, and I have all the time in the world. I am here to receive the self-care ritual of the sacred baths.

I can do this visualization anywhere at any time I feel like a self-care ritual. I also do this when I wash my hands. I imagine that the water and the soap are deeply purifying my entire being right through the palms of my hands. I imagine pulling in the mineral rich water through my hands and my wrists and even as the water swirls down the drain I imagine it as crystal clear water being taken through ancient tunnels, purifying again as it goes.

I also do this with vacations. I visualize fully a vacation experience. Remember the brain doesn't know the difference if the experience is an inner or an outer experience. So, if my mind and body need to feel like they have been on vacation to reduce my stress levels and raise my happiness levels then I am all in! There is no additional cost to imagining more great self-care experiences, so feel free to be abundant in your imagination.

The Self-Care Breathing Practice (Breathing/Words)

This practice of fully conscious breathing is how we began our journey, breathing from the four parts of our breath.

Inhale, Retain, Exhale, and Pause.

As a foundational practice, this breathing becomes our formal operating system for the body as well as the mind and we call it our Magical Moment. We breathe in through the nose and out through the nose for this practice. Inhale, Retain, Exhale, Pause.

Inhale easefully and deeply.

Now **retain** your breath, hold your breath for a second or two but allow this retention to be its own full part of the breath, so hold just a moment or so but let the retention have its space.

Exhale easefully and deeply, take your time and exhale completely.

Pause for as long as is natural for you. You do not need to force your inhales as they will come naturally. Just hang out in the pause at the end of your exhale until your inhale comes.

Do as many Magical Moment breaths as flow naturally over the course of one minute to become familiar with this gentle pattern. Then expand to two minutes, then three and so on. Breathe this way for as long as feels good to you.

Extra: Add a self-care blessing to your Magical Moment breath. As you inhale think to yourself, "my body, I love you" as you exhale think to yourself, "my body, I thank you."

The Self-Care Physical Practice (Physical/Actions)
Our movement practice to anchor Self-Care into the body is a simple yoga exercise that can be done standing or seated.

Begin with your hands at your heart, palms together in prayer position, gently connecting thumbs to your heart space in the centre of your chest.

Pause here and connect to your breath, when you feel ready to move, and in harmony with your inhale, raise your arms out to the sides and up over head, as high as they go naturally. Retain your breath in this position, arms up. When your exhale comes at its natural pace lower your arms, hands back to heart centre. Again, inhale and raise your arms overhead, exhale hands back to your heart. Continue to move in this way, establishing a harmonious connection with your breath and your body.

Adding on: Inhale, raise your arms out to the sides and up over head and when your exhale comes begin to fold forward as far as you go naturally, hang out in the pause at the end of your exhale. Then as your inhale comes naturally, bend your knees a little, press into your feet and come up slowly. Then follow through, raising your arms up. Retain your breath and when your exhale comes naturally take your hands back to heart centre. Repeat this gentle flow establishing a harmonious connection with your breath and your body.

Work your way up to 8, and from there you can do as many as makes you happy. Make it your focus to move in harmony with your natural breathing pattern; inhale, retain, exhale, and pause. Some days you will be a little faster, some days a little slower, just maintain a collaboration between your breath and movement.

Never force your movements during the practices. Simply meet your body wherever it is at each time you do the exercises and you will see that it will change from day to day. As well, as you become stronger and more flexible you will notice changes. I understand for some of you when I say work your way up to 8, it will seem too basic for you since you are physically capable of doing 108. What a blessing that you are so strong and flexible. Sister, so go ahead and do as many as you love!

This yoga flow is great for re-establishing harmony of breath and body. It cultivates co-ordination, increases our energy levels, and strengthens and stretches the spine. It maintains our range of motion in our shoulders and brings more blood flow to all the moving parts of our body, including the spine. Compressing the abdomen and organs on the forward folds helps maintain the healthy organs and cleanse our system. Moving our body in harmony with our breath retrains us to use our energy in a more balanced way, increasing our energy, maintaining our energy longer.

Chapter Two

THE SECOND SACRED RESPONSIBILITY: RISE AND SHINE

Stepping onto a brand-new path is difficult, but not more difficult than remaining in a situation which is not nurturing to the whole woman.

—*Maya Angelou*

I have exciting news for you! Shining into our greatness is a by-product of Self-Care. Yep! We have already begun to expose more of our light when our self-care practices begin to build our foundation of a healthy body, healthy mind and healthy heart. When we are feeling even just ten percent happier, healthier and livelier we are simply more vibrant, shinier!

We start by showing up in our life *choosing* to shine. We actually have the capability to move our lives in so many directions and Rise and Shine as the second Sacred Responsibility tell us to do just that, to lean into our lives be fully present, participate like it is the best day of your life. And, yes, even when we are challenged, finding the strength to rise up. We rise and shine for ourselves first because we are worthy of a life well-lived, and second because there is always someone watching us as their mentoring example of how a life well lived can look. There is always someone learning from observing us and noticing how we manage ourselves in our day to day lives. Usually, we are not even aware of who that person is. May we inspire those who are observing us by being our most authentic selves and encourage them by example to be their most authentic selves also.

Choose to Rise and Shine

Rise and Shine, ladies, because we are making history for ourselves right now! Each one of us in this moment. Here, Now, and Together. We are in a position to write the story of an entire adult life for ourselves, to write the story of our lives that will leave the greatest impact on our families, in our communities and in our overall story. I believe that with every thought word and action we make during this Third Act Movement we are leaving a gorgeous imprint of light for future women to warm themselves in and inspire them to accept the torch from us when we enter our fourth act—the next book!

Although history is of the past, it is not created in the past, it is created in the present moment. The wisdom of the Dalai Lama reminds us that:

There are only two days in the year that nothing can be done, one is called yesterday, and the other is called tomorrow. So today is the right day to love, believe, do, and mostly live.

And, may I add, take Sacred Responsibility

As we begin accepting the Sacred Responsibility to Rise and Shine in our lives we are taking full responsibility for the legacy we will leave once we depart from this life. When we Rise and Shine in our lives each day, we no longer see ourselves as simply products of our past, but pioneering souls of our future. Once we embrace the mindset that every thought, word, and action create the imprint we leave behind, we realize that how we contribute to the story of our own legacy is completely up to us! The imprint and story we leave is created by our choices and by the decisions we make in the present moment. The choice to Rise and Shine, to show up every day in our lives like we matter and that our happiness matters, our vitality matters and our relationships matter. The present moment is like the fertile soil we plant our legacy seeds in. When nurtured by taking sacred responsibility to Rise and Shine these creative seeds can grow into our rich story of a woman in her third act, who lived a life understanding that it is a Sacred Responsibility to Rise and Shine, to choose to create meaning and to locate inspiration each day. *Your* first chapter begins now!

Igniting Our Passion

We now ignite our passion to *consciously* Rise and Shine writing our new story with every thought, word and action. We are the Writers, Directors and Producers of our own play, our own plan and our own legacy.

Our legacy is in the making with or without our conscious participation. Moments in time will continue to unfold and how we choose to be present within this unfolding is completely up to us. We have the idea of being the writers of our third act story and we have a starting point as we are here together in this present moment. But now what? Where to go from here? What will the future fiery and fabulous women in their third act be reading about us and which of our stories will they tell?

Everything you do counts for-ever. You are an expression of the whole process of creation; you are a co-creator.
—Barbara Marx Hubbard

First: We get all fired up about it! Get turned on about it! We ignite the sacred fire of passion in our hearts. We get ourselves into a state of coherence.

Second: We ask ourselves the three questions of a Sacred Woman who takes Sacred Responsibility to Rise and Shine in her life and thus in her legacy.

1. Are my thoughts, words and actions in alignment with my third act story?
2. Are my thoughts, words and actions in alignment with my legacy?
3. Are my thoughts, words and actions in alignment with my happiness?

If you answer yes to any of these questions you are hon-ouring the Second Sacred Responsibility Rise and Shine.

Relationships
One of the most satisfying places to Rise and Shine is in our relationships. All of them. Your intimate relationships, your family relationships, your friendships, the relation-ships you have with the natural world and your relation-ship with yourself. When we live from a place of taking Sa-cred Responsibility to Rise and Shine in our relationships

we get to ask ourselves new questions, and feel free to add more to our list.

1. Do my thoughts, words, and actions contribute to an elevated and shiny relationship?
2. Do my thoughts, words, and actions contribute to kindness in this relationship?
3. Do my thoughts, words, and actions contribute to respect in this relationship?
4. Do my thoughts, words, and actions contribute to understanding in this relationship?
5. Do my thoughts, words, and actions contribute to happiness in this relationship?
6. Do my thoughts, words, and actions contribute to healthy boundaries in this relationship?

These questions are to inspire you to be active in the way you relate to others. It is particularly important to be inspired in our intimate relationships, our relationships with our partners, our family members and our nearest and dearest friends. It is our plan to thrive in our third act, and we are setting the stage by taking Sacred Responsibility for the quality of our relationships. And yes, many times it will be us that makes the first move in this area because we are inspired to include healthy, happy relationships in our life well-lived. It is absolutely our pleasure to lead in this area and be the change we want to see in our relationships.

Shiny, Elevated Relationships

We can all relate to the feelings we get when we spend time with someone we really enjoy. The conversations and activities are so interesting, uplifting, and fun that the time just seems to fly. We are at a time in our lives that we can cultivate even deeper connections with the people in our lives who stoke our fire. We have a little more time and a lot more interest in experiencing our relationships from a place of sacred responsibility.

Go ahead, Rise and Shine here, become more understanding, become a deeper listener, become more open to the subtleties of those close to you who are making shifts and changes in their lives also. This is important, as we take sacred responsibility to write our new passionate life stories, as well as engage in our practices, we will create change in us that connects us more deeply to our ourselves and the way we wish to relate to our most intimate people. We will respond from a more interested and passionate place than we may have done in our past, and we also we will know exactly how we want to spend our time and our efforts in our relationships now.

As we are developing these traits through taking sacred responsibility for our thoughts, words, and actions we will be changing our environment, both inner and outer. Our personal environment will shift. Others in our lives will feel and see we are coming from a refreshed perspective and, as we learn to "hold" the vibration of our practices in day to day life, it will give those we are in relationship with permission to do the same. Our commitment to our practice of taking the Sacred Responsibility to Rise and Shine will be the example set.

Rise and Shine: The Heart Centered Expression of You

There is a newer field of study called neurocardiology and these scientists are discovering that the heart is more functionally sophisticated then had been previously discussed in the scientific circles over the last few hundred years (the ancients knew full well the power of the heart, we just took a bit of a nap in this area until recently).

Our practices of a mind, body, heart connection/balance provide a path towards what the HeartMath Institute teaches us is Coherence—a state of optimal functioning.

I am including the link to the full article on their site in the resources section as it is interesting and totally supportive of what we are setting out to accomplish for ourselves as we rise and shine. I have been fascinated by their research for years and if you have not heard of HeartMath yet, you are in for a treat!

HeartMath shares over twenty-five years of scientific research on the psychophysiology of stress, emotions, and the interactions between the heart and brain. There are over three hundred peer-reviewed or independent research studies published about the beneficial outcomes for us when we are in a state of coherence.

Not only do they have the years of research behind them, but they have developed technology to measure the frequencies we operate from and show them to us on a screen. We can watch our frequency change right before our eyes as we implement exercises that bring coherence into the mind, heart and body.

The practices of The Eight Sacred Responsibilities are our particular path to living from a state of coherence. I have put our practices to the test (repeatedly) on the Heart-Math technology which I have in my office. My personal research has concluded that when we engage in the practices laid out for us in this book to work with, play with, and be supported by, we indeed will find ourselves in a state of Coherence. Cool eh!

Relating to the young adults in our lives

I have been thinking about this and would like to get the conversation flowing in our community. I have been hearing a lot of negative conversation directed at our Millennials, our young people born in the 80's and 90's. I have heard some serious conversations about an overall feeling of entitlement, that this generation lacks a work ethic and all kinds of less than loving chat about the people who will be our care-givers in our fourth act.

In my own experience, I have incredibly fun, strong, smart caring young people in my life and they have like-hearted friends. These are Millennials who happily enjoy being with older people and take responsibility for their share of the work around the home. They are innovative, interesting, respect nature and I could go on.

So, I am not honestly100% tuned into the harsher conversations this generation seems to have directed their way. But I understand it is a great concern to many who are having this Millennial experience, so I would like our community to support those with this concern in their hearts.

As I have been thinking about the movement of disappointment in the Millennials it prompted the question: what if it is our work in the realms of Sacred Responsibility that sets just the kind of example it takes to turn these concerns around?

As we take Sacred Responsibility for ourselves we will do less blaming and shaming and more inspiring and encouraging. By developing our responsibility for our own happiness and our ability to enjoy life and relationships fully, our young people will be mentored by us. Like all of our relationships, whether they be our intimate relationships with our partners, or those with our children and grandchildren or the relationships with our closest friends, we are the ones stepping into Sacred Responsibility. It is our pleasure to make the first move.

Trust that with beautiful, respectful mentorship our younger generations will Rise and Shine and be greater then we could have guessed! May we lead by shiny example.

Our Second Sacred Practice

Our Daily Statement
Today I open myself fully to living a sacred life, I call in now the people, places and things that lift me up, light me up and hold me up as the accountable, responsible and authentic woman I am here to be. And so it is.

**The Rise and Shine Imagination Practice
(Imagining/Thoughts)**

As we begin to look forward to Rising and Shining in our third act, we use all the superpowers we have in our imagination and we start to set our intention each day of what we want to present to the world. So, we send a Sacred Package forward to the end of our day with this intention.

Start by making a conscious decision about how you want to show up today and what you want to show to the world, to your family, friends, and to your community. Now prepare to send your package forward.

TIP: This is something you could write in your journal daily.

Once you have decided how you want to present yourself today, imagine now you send an energetic package or template of that ahead to the end of your day. Stay with me here, this is a powerful exercise in self-actualization and we are going to understand it slowly and together.

Let me give you a couple of examples of how I use the Sacred Package. I do this shortly after waking up, either in bed or as I am brushing my teeth, but within the first half hour to hour of waking up.

I think happily of how I would like to present myself today, what I would like to show to the world as I move around in my day. Today, as I think of all the possibilities, I decide I would like to show the part of me that is a deep listener. Today I will talk a little less and enjoy heart-centred listening with the people I come across during my day. I want anyone I connect with today to know that part of me. I want people to feel that they have been heard by me. This could be in person, on the phone or any of the ways we communicate like email or texting, etc. But today I show up as a deep listener.

Then I send that energy in my Sacred Package ahead of me to the end of my day as if it has already happened. Now I just get to enjoy the journey of my day and I'll join up with the package tonight when I go to bed.

I also send Sacred Packages forward when I travel, for example as soon as the plane ticket is bought, or the plan made to travel somewhere, I begin to visualize my return. I send a Sacred Package forward in thoughts and visualization. I see myself arriving back home, happy and excited to tell my travel stories. I picture myself coming into my apartment after my journey, putting my feet up, scrolling through my photos, snuggling my cat and feeling amazing about my adventure. I send it forward that the experience concludes with me happy, healthy and safe.

Now bring to your mind what aspects of yourself you would love to present today.

Give yourself a few moments to visualize and feel these aspects of yourself in action today.

Take your time, visualize for as long as you like.

And when you feel like you've really got it, go ahead and imagine now that the energy of how you want to show up and what aspects of yourself you would like to share with the world today get packaged up into a beautiful Sacred Package.

Imagine sending that package forward to the end of your day.

See the package land in your bed on your pillow where

you will meet up with it later. You can even use your hands and physically place your imagined Sacred Package on your pillow.

Your package may look like a gift, it may look like a sparkly paper airplane, it may look like you have thrown a golden baseball forward to the end of your day.

Use your imagination and make your Sacred Package fabulous.

Now go about your day knowing that it is so.

Once you send out your completed Sacred Package, say to yourself 'and so it is'. Then go about your day happily. This is meant to be fun, and to begin to get us tuned into exactly how we want to show up for ourselves and others and begin to see it as a done deal. We are dreaming into reality the full expression of our fiery and fabulous selves. Conceive it, believe it, achieve it.

Rise and Shine for the difficult day

We use our imagination practices for empowered playful thoughts that turn into our empowered and playful words that turn into our empowered and playful actions. All in support of increasing our life force and to assist us in building new neuro pathways. There will be some days that you would rather bury yourself under the covers than Rise and Shine, this is part of the tapestry of our lives and, sisters, we've got this. In our self-respecting acts of compassion, we have an imagination practice for the painful days.

There is an audio recording of this exercise to support you, so you can relax deeply into this healing visualization. Enter the Sacred Portal for our recordings at www.reachyogalifestyle.ca

Make yourself comfortable, sitting or lying down.

Connect to the feeling you have now that is holding you back from Rising and Shining today.

You may be in pain over loss, you may feel deep disappointment, or it's anger or shame.

Whatever it is that is your overwhelming feeling right now, just go into it, feel it, sit with it and breathe. Breathe deeply in and out of your nose. Take your time, you are not alone.

Begin to imagine that you see yourself as a child.

Notice what age you are in your imagination.

Imagine you see yourself as a little girl in a playground.

Notice the slides and swing sets, notice the weather and the sounds.

Imagine, as you see yourself as a little girl, that you can tell that she in pain.

Observe her for a few breaths, notice what she is wearing, what kind of shoes she has on, what her hair looks like. Simply observe you as a little girl.

You get up from your observation bench and start to walk towards her.

You see she is alone, and she is not playing with the other children.

As you walk towards her, you can feel so much love filling your heart for her dear sweet soul who is in so much pain.

As you get closer, she sees you walking towards her and she recognises you immediately and you see in her face that she is relieved you have shown up for her today.

When you reach her, kneel so you can be at her level and take her hand.

Take a few deep breaths. Take your time, let her cry if she needs to cry.

Imagine she lets you hug her, wrap your arms around her and let her feel that you are here for her, that you are not going to leave her.

Breathe and take all the time here you like.

Ask her if she would like to tell you what is hurting her so much today.

Now listen, listen until she feels completely heard, heard by your adult-self.

Breathe with her and listen.

When she is finished telling you about her pain, ask her if there is anything she would like you to do for her.

Listen to what she needs from you and give that to her.

If she needs you to hear her pain, be a deep listener for her.

If she needs you to protect her, do so with all your heart.

If she needs you to tell her she is safe, go ahead and tell her.

Imagine your adult-self helping your little girl feel anything she needs to feel, safe, heard, and protected by you right now.

Tell her that you will always be here for her. Tell her that you will never leave her and that she can count on you always.

Now imagine taking what you just told her and wrapping it up in a Sacred Package. Your words and your feelings wrapped up into a beautiful Sacred Package. Make it as pretty and as fun as you know she would love.

Now give her the Sacred Package. Let her know she can

unwrap it anytime she needs to feel or hear the words you have spoken to her today. The package can be opened millions of times, as it never loses any of its power.

Imagine that you wipe the tears from her cheeks, and you both stand up and you take her hand and begin to walk together.

Imagine as you walk and talk, that with each step you see her begin to become a playful child again.

You can see her light shining from her eyes again and her smile and you know she feels heard by you and safe to start her day from this point.

Use this imagination practice anytime you need, sisters. Feel supported by all of us reading this book. Feel the strength of your adult-self standing up strongly for the little girl inside of you. The little girl inside each of us is incredibly wise, incredibly resilient, and full of creativity and play. Let your adult-self stand beside her as a wise guardian. Take care of her as you would any child, anyone vulnerable, anyone in pain.

The Rise and Shine Breathing Practice (Breathing/Words)

Our Practice is to anchor Rise and Shine as a Sacred Responsibility into our body and our energy field. This a practice of fully conscious breathing is just like we began our journey, breathing from the four parts of our breath. Inhale, Retain, Exhale, and Pause. In our Rise and Shine Power Breath we add energy to this breathing pattern.

This Power Breath has three inhales through the nose and out through the nose.

Then three in through the nose and out through the *mouth*.

We would say 3 nose-nose and 3 nose-mouth.

Continue to breathe in the same pattern as you have been in the Magical Moment breath, inhale, retain, exhale, and pause. But now we exaggerate the inhale and exhale.

Tip: *Blow your nose before beginning this exercise.*

Our inhale is a big sniff (yes, there is sound) and our exhale out the nose is equally as strong. Big sniff inhale, retain, big sniff out exhale.

We do not need to rush it, make it smooth and even, but a powerful sniff in and a sniff out.

On the exhale, you can slightly constrict the muscles in your throat and push the air out by squeezing your belly muscles at the same time as your exhale.

There will be sound when you inhale with your big sniff in, and sound on your exhale when you press out all of the air.

Three breaths nose-nose. In through the nose and out through the nose.

Now, three breaths nose-mouth.

Take a big sniff in through the nose and exhale through the mouth make a round shape with your mouth as if you were saying Ho.

Big sniff in through the nose, big Ho out through the mouth.

Do three of each to start.

Work your way up to three sets of three over a few

weeks. Remember we have all kinds of time, a full adult life of time to work our way up to three sets of three.

Even though this is a power breath it is still long and luxurious.

Full breaths, deep breaths and take your time on your exhale, gently squeezing our all the air with a squeeze to your third chakra. The solar plexus area between your bellybutton and your lower breastbone.

This is the first exercise in our practice that starts to build the strength of the solar plexus, preparing us to be strong, ready and resilient for whatever may come along that tries to take away our personal power.

This is a deep cleansing breathing practice that in yoga is given in a more advanced setting. I know it seems simple, but I am going to strongly suggest if you are new to breathing exercises that you work with this one in a seated position until you become comfortable with your body's response.

This power breathing exercise helps to strengthen your lungs, energize you and settle you, strong and peaceful.

The Rise and Shine Physical Practice (Physical/Actions)

We continue to work with the strength of the solar plexus, third chakra and the power residing in the abdomen. We are cultivating strength from the core out. As we build our strength and coordination this movement will strengthen us from our feet to our solar plexus as well as build upper body strength. Here are a few options depending on your level of energy and strength:

Level One: We use the exhale as our engine to run this exercise, it will be our power centre. To begin you can be seated, standing, or laying down. Start by taking a full belly breath on your inhale, then as you exhale squeeze your belly button towards your spine, again inhale full belly and exhale squeezing your belly button towards your spine, inhale full belly breath, exhale squeezing your belly button towards your spine.

Continue breathing this way for about a minute starting to strengthen the centre or the core of your body. You can even begin to engage all the muscles from your pubic bone to your sternum, activating all the muscles that support your spine and the strength of your abdomen. If your energy levels are low today this can be the complete exercise. Continue breathing full belly and work on squeezing all the muscles of your abdomen toward your spine.

Level Two: Assume a seated or standing position and continue with the same breathing in, full belly, but this time as you inhale raise your arms. As you exhale, make slightly squeezed fists and pull your elbows down towards your rib cage as you squeeze your belly.

Inhale and raise your arms. As you exhale, make slightly squeezed fists and pull your elbows down towards your rib cage as you squeeze your belly. Squeeze your underarm muscles when you bring your elbows close to your ribcage.

Continue for one full minute and on your last exhale lay your hands over your heart, close your eyes, and breathe.

Level Three. Start from a standing position, feet a comfortable hip width apart (your feet are as wide as you need so that your knees feel strong and protected from the stress of too much pressure).

Inhale and raise your arms. As you exhale, make slightly squeezed fists and pull your elbows towards your rib cage as you squeeze your belly and bend into your knees slightly or deeply whatever is good for you today.

From your squat position, press strongly into your feet, inhale come up and reach up. Exhale, make small fists and pull your elbows towards your ribs and sink into your squat again.

Level Four. On the days you feel high energy and strength, we add on a holding position. Feet are a comfortable hip-width apart. Inhale and raise your arms. As you exhale, make slightly squeezed fists and pull your elbows towards your rib cage as you squeeze your belly and bend into your knees deeply and comfortably.

Do this sequence three times.

On the third time, hold in your squat.

You can go ahead and extend your arms out in front or slightly above.

Hold for three deep breaths.

On your third exhale, bring your elbows back to your ribs, hands to your heart and inhale.

Then use the power of your exhale to press yourself up to standing. Hands over your heart relax and breathe.

Tip: *Be mindful of your knees.*

Yes, we are building strength and endurance and we are also cultivating alignment. If your knees feel any pain, stop, take a break and readjust. You can even begin by using something supportive like a table or counter to hold onto just to find the best position for your knees.

Never force your movements during the practices, simply meet your body wherever it is at each time you do the exercises and you will see that it will change from day to day, as well, as you become stronger and more flexible you will notice changes.

I understand that for some of you when I say work your way up to 8 it will seem too basic since you are physically capable of doing many more and what a blessing you are so strong and flexible, sister. Go ahead and do as many as you love!

You are worthy, you are powerful, and you are strong.

Chapter Three

The Third Sacred Responsibility: Know Yourself

You need to learn to select your thoughts just the same way you select your clothes every day. This is a power you can cultivate.

—Elizabeth Gilbert

And I mean ***really*** know yourself. Understand every response, every reaction, every part of your body and every part of your life. Know it, own it and implement your plan of thriving in your third act. Know yourself as a Sacred Responsibility. It is our sacred responsibility to know ourselves so that we may thrive in this life by shifting the energy of the things that keep us stuck so we can shine in the things that make us shimmer with life-force. Knowing our self is self-empowerment.

Let's face it, sisters. Knowing ourselves *is* power. When we know what increases and decreases our life-force we are empowered and at this time in our lives we are making it our sacred responsibility to increase our life force, not decrease it.

How would you expect to have the best time of your life if you don't even know what you love to do most?

How could you have your most open mind if you don't know where you are stuck in judgement? How could you have the most open heart if you don't even know what makes you most happy? How could you take responsibility for fabulous body health if you don't even know what actions make you feel better or worse? Get to know yourself intimately.

Keep the wisdom, toss the judgment
Our thoughts begin in our head, then come out of our mouths and show up in our actions and inevitably express themselves in our bodies. Tending to our thoughts, words and actions like a fascinated explorer makes the journey exciting and decreases self-judgement in the process which is great training ground for not judging others.

Over the course of your exploration, and taking the Sacred Responsibility to Know Yourself, you are going to come to terms with how you have treated yourself in the past. You may be surprised to realize how long you have been active in a behaviour that is on your list of, "things that don't make me feel good".

Let's treat it as if we are digging up a buried treasure, let it come up and out. When something comes up for you like this, go ahead and take a moment to ask yourself, "what the hell was I thinking?" But inquire only to know yourself better as you move forward in Self-Care.

The issue with behaviours that are no longer serving us is that we don't know until we know. And we are way too old to be judging ourselves for anything about our past. We are creating our revised third act plan, our vision of how we truly want to feel in our lives.

Living from an old program, our family stories

Sometimes we will carry stories of our family in such a tight grip that it becomes nearly impossible to penetrate the actual origins of the story, "because that is the way we do it this family." Period. Questioning a family belief rarely even comes to mind for most of us. There is an unconscious agreement we have in our families to protect our story. Then all it takes is one pioneering soul to come along and ask, "why?"

Enter my version of The Pot Roast Story:

A young woman is preparing a pot roast while her friend looks on. She cuts off both ends of the roast, seasons it and puts it in the pan.

"Why do you cut off the ends?" her friend asks.

"I don't know. My mother always did it that way and I learned how to cook it from her."

Her friend's question made her curious about her pot roast preparation. During her next visit home, she asked her mother, "How do you cook a pot roast?"

Her mother proceeded to explain and added, "You cut off both ends, season it, put it in the pot and then in the oven."

"Why do you cut off the ends?" the daughter asked.

Baffled, the mother offered, "That's how my mother did it and I learned it from her!"

Her daughter's inquiry made the mother think more about the pot roast preparation. When she next visited her mother she asked, "Mom, how do you cook a pot roast?"

"Well, you prepare it with spices, cut off both ends and put it in the pot."

She asked her mom, "But why do you cut off the ends?"

"Well, the roasts were always bigger than the pot that we had back then. I had to cut off the ends to fit it into the pot that I owned"

The "why" of the family story was that simple…

Knowing Yourself in Relationships

Until we make knowing ourselves a priority, to really look at what lifts us up and what brings us down, we will keep on doing the same things to exhaustion. When the plan is to rock our third act, we need to clean house in all areas of our life and it is not always going to be pretty. Occasionally we are going to open a jar from the back of the fridge and gag. But don't forget that there was a point when that festering jar of slime mattered to you, which may be a metaphor for some old relationships too.

If we can get really honest with ourselves and deeply compassionate, it will be much easier to see when we are bringing an outdated family belief into our third act relationships. I watch many couples (and close friends) struggle in their relationships because they don't realize they are fighting for a certain belief that came from a passed-down family program that most times doesn't even apply to their modern experience.

Let me put this way, have you ever thought for a moment, "oh my God, I'm my Mother!"? Then you have more clarity in this area of how we naturally mimic the ones who raised us, including the beliefs that were passed down to them while they were being raised.

Knowing Yourself as a Sacred Responsibility is the key

to freeing yourself up to live your own interesting life and living richly within your relationships. Get to know what your belief is, and what is someone else's belief you have unconsciously adopted.

Rebranding in Relationships

Anyone who knows me knows that I find kindness hot! I prefer rebranding in relationships that seem to be stuck, and I love the power and maturity that can be found in getting through something that seems like it is a deal breaker. No one really wants to hurt another person and when we get hurt it is more likely that we have a past pain rising up and inserting itself into the situation. Know yourself, know what you truly believe and know what comes from an old program.

It is a natural way of the mind to continually scan all of our past experiences and apply them to our current experiences. We could look at it as the way we can find our equilibrium in our lives, how we make sense of things, to understand our relationship to our environment. Our mind will search in our stored data and present it as evidence.

If we are not willing to enjoy and cultivate our own growth, change, and maturity, we will have a hard time seeing the opportunity to do this in our relationships, and it will become very difficult to maintain a healthy, honest relationship. We absolutely must take sacred responsibility to get to know the areas where we need to grow, mature, and make changes so that we can thrive in fulfilling relationships. There is absolutely nothing that can bring us more happiness then fulfilling friendships.

Go ahead, try and think of something else more fulfilling than your relationships with others, then think about that thing without anyone to share it with, ever. A fiery and fabulous woman in her third act honours her relationships like the treasures they are. Go for it, ladies! Bring your most loving, honest, kind and vulnerable self to your relationships and enjoy each other fully. People are beautiful, people are sacred, and always remember people have feelings. Be kind, it's hot!

You: Then and Now

I have a pair of white baby boots hanging just above my coat closet at home and every day I see them. They have been there for years. My mom gave them to me one day and I didn't find any significance in the boots at the time or for many years after. But there did come a time, not all that long ago, when I saw them in a whole new light.

I began to see those boots as a symbol of my growth and maturity. For so many years they were simply a cute reminder of me as a baby. As the story goes, I walked very early on so the shoes would give me a laugh when they caught my eye, reminding me that I've been on the move right from the start.

Now when I look at those boots I see my potential. I see endless possibilities for myself and they remind me now that there is so much more to come. The amount of life experience I've had since the time those shoes fit is quite incredible to me. The places I've been, the people I've met, the things that I have learned and all the rich experiences I have had in this life so far shine from the shoes.

It is exciting for me to be reminded that I am no longer

that person. I'm not the eight-month-old child walking for the first time but a wise and loving woman who has left thousands of footprints over many parts of the world. The shoes have been with me for so many years and wherever I lived I have always hammered a nail above the coat closet and hung these baby boots there.

Originally, they were a funny symbol pointing people to the coat cupboard, but as I've matured their symbolism has matured with me. They now represent so much more, and I think I have an understanding now why people bronze their baby shoes!

A very easy way to start this process of getting to know yourself and understanding your growth is to look at a pair of shoes or a piece of clothing from your childhood. If you don't have anything like that available to you, look at a childhood photo. If you are unable to find something of your own, use something that you still have from your children's past.

You can see quite clearly that the shoes or sweater no longer fit, that the writing in a birthday card a child made for you is not the way they write as an adult. And we don't force them to wear the old shoes or sweaters that no longer fit. We let ourselves and others grow up.

With that in mind, can we stop holding ourselves and others so tightly gripped to past stories and experiences? We are not that person anymore, but we can certainly enjoy the journey that we have made to this point and feel excited about the journey ahead filled with our infinite potential still as a creative force in our lives. Make space to know yourself by watching how you create your new stories, not relive your past ones.

Know yourself and how you respond to life

Let's face it, giving our happiness as much consideration as we give our disappointment is going to take an overhaul of the way we think. It calls for a complete 'renovation' of the quality of our thoughts, words, and actions from this moment forward, starting with how we respond to life.

When living in sacred responsibility we take on the joyous task of being responsible for our happiness, for our joy, for our connection to others, and for our gratitude for the absolute treat it is to be alive.

We no longer point fingers and blame others for our dissatisfaction in any areas of our life, even if we believe it is their fault. We no longer *make* it anyone else's responsibility to make us happy because we do that for ourselves. Let us be open to the notion that when we shift our thoughts words and actions towards greater clarity and happiness we may just inspire those closest to us to do the same. We take full responsibility and we rise to the occasion, very like a Phoenix from the ashes, because we are both fiery and fabulous.

The mythology of the Phoenix rising from the ashes is a great symbol to inspire us and to use as a template for seeing ourselves overcoming adversity—even the death of something that we loved or deeply identified with. This Greek myth tell us that the Phoenix is a bird that had a life span of hundreds of years. At conclusion of this long life, the Phoenix with its fiery plumage returns to its nest, where both bird and nest are reduced to ashes in a fabulous show of flames. And, from the ashes the new life is born. So, it is a story of change, rebirth, liberation, new life.

A Change of Perspective

Some hard truth: the people who we want to blame for our lack of joy, the ones who said or did something (or many things) to disappoint us are usually the ones who need more understanding, more patience and more love. And, many times we have to be more understanding, patient and loving from afar. While we are taking responsibility for our thoughts, words, and actions we are beginning to gently and lovingly liberate ourselves from our life's sorrows that can bury themselves deeply into our cells and keep us from living fully and passionately. Part of knowing ourselves and of living passionately, is fully feeling all that the experiences have brought us.

Little by little we find the wisdom in the sorrow, we begin to tell the story differently and we trust that our happiness does not depend on anything but our choice to see things differently, for our own peace. In that, it is an act of loving-kindness for all involved. *A Course in Miracles* (Dr. Helen Schucman) teaches us that a miracle is a change in perspective. That seems so empowering to me and a beautiful message of taking Sacred Responsibility for the way we see things.

Getting to know the new you!

Sometimes the first stage of becoming the next great version of ourselves is by recognizing the parts of us that we no longer identify with. I was having lunch with a girlfriend and she was saying how her husband was going on about how great she was at being on top of everything, and how she can take care of business better than anyone he knows and on and on about how fabulous and efficient she is.

How nice to receive all of that praise right? Yet she found her response to his enthusiasm over her ability to multitask, read the fine print, and cook Super Bowl chili all at the same time was, "I'm not that person anymore."

He said, "Oh sure you are you are so good at…"

And she said, "Honey, look at me. I am not that person anymore, that was 25 years of being that, and I am happily not that person anymore." She said it calmly and kindly.

She said he paused and said, "Wow, ok yeah, I can see what you are saying."

Fabulous lunch conversation for a woman who is writing a book on rewriting our story! I share this because I loved that she didn't need to stomp her feet and scream about how she wants things to be different at this time in her life. She didn't have to blame anyone for holding her to a life she now considered a memory. She simply stated that she is not that person anymore in a kind way and had no feeling she needed to make any excuses or explain herself.

She took sacred responsibility for her leaving her "old self" to great memories *and* she expressed to her husband that she was operating a new way now!

I did ask her, "Well if you are not that person anymore, who are you now?"

She thought for a moment, laughed, and said, "I haven't decided yet."

The ultimate in "being okay" with not knowing yourself while you are getting to Know Yourself!

I am always so happy to hear the stories of women who are transforming their lives in a way that gives them and those around them peace and in ways that maintain their energy levels. It's hard to be a fabulous Phoenix rising from your nest of ashes if someone douses your flames with a lack of understanding that you have a desire to shift or change something about yourself.

I love this story for many reasons but something else that stands out is that the things she said "she was not" anymore were things that are great attributes, these things were compliments and her partner's observations of how fantastic he thought she was. I loved the power in choosing not to be "that person" anymore even when "that person" is awesome!

Change because it excites you

Sisters, I want us all to lean in on this one and really hear it. We do not have to choose to change because we don't like something in our lives, we can choose to change because we are happily complete with something in our lives. We can choose to change because it excites us.

Can you hear it in that way? I do not need to leave my job because I hate it, I can leave my job because I created a more fitting opportunity elsewhere. I don't have to stop eating junk because it is well...junk. I can stop eating junk because I have discovered other yummy things that raise my energy. I do not have to move across town because I hate my neighbors. I move across town because I found more like-hearted neighbors in another area.

I bring these examples up because we are starting to live from an energy of wisdom now. We do not have to wait until we are frustrated and angry with something in our lives in order to make a change. When we take sacred responsibility for our happiness we see the signs long before a situation gets so big that we find ourselves "hating" a part of our lives. We are so tuned into what raises our energy and what depletes it that we see the red flags. We see the signs that change is our best choice well before it gets to a point of hate.

This is one of the blessings of life over fifty. We change things in our inner and outer environments because we love to, not because we "have to". That is an old way of connecting with change and we take sacred responsibility for our change, which in itself makes us happy. We are prepared to be challenged at times, and we are building our resilience for just those times, because change will come whether we plan it in advance or wait for it to smack us upside the head. Change is a guarantee.

Ladies, I see our sacred journey together to be exciting and filled with change and growth, and that has very little to do with changing because we dislike things in our lives, or about ourselves. Occasionally things like that will rise to the surface. Heck, we have been living this life for some time now so some of the dust bunnies are bound to come out from under the couch and we can thank them for their dusty wisdom and burn them to ashes.

Moving forward together, we steer our hearts in new directions, into the mystery that living from our most authentic self will surely reveal.

Know Yourself, Challenge Your Negativity

It baffles me how easily we can loop into a negative spin sending ourselves down a rabbit hole of disappointment. Going from a moment of ease just walking down the street to utter disappointment in the blink of an eye, or more fitting, in the shift of the mind.

We are amazing human beings who can go from joy to distain in the snap of a finger and we do it with gusto! And then we get really into it and before we know it we have decided everyone is against us, no one can be trusted with our hearts, and we are not worthy of respect. Top that off with your wallet dumping all of your change on the ground at the bus stop and it's a perfect human storm of total disappointment. And it's not even lunch time yet!

What I will propose to all of us using this book, *The Eight Sacred Responsibilities* is that together, we challenge ourselves. Challenge ourselves to observe from a renewed perspective of sacred responsibility those shifts in our mind that take us down the rabbit hole of disappointment and rewire our operating system so that more often than not we are coming from a place of balance. I will warn you—it's not going to happen overnight.

If I handed out guitars right now and said, "We are all going to play *Stairway to Heaven*", most of us would need some practice time. We would have questions, need to organize ourselves a bit (or a lot!) but it wouldn't happen with a snap of a finger. We would need a bit of time to get into harmony with each other.

So, we can look at the areas in our life where we have a desire to shift, change and grow as a learning experience just as if we are learning to play a complicated song on a guitar. One note at a time, that will turn into a chord, turning into a second chord with each step becoming a satisfying thirst for doing things differently.

And yep… occasionally it will get complicated because change is made of rubber. It stretches us and then we bounce back to our original mindsets. Then it stretches us a little further and when we bounce back we don't go quite as far into our old stories. We are setting ourselves up to thrive in a brand-new story, one that is so interesting it is like we are reading a fascinating novel about a strong woman explorer. But instead of reading about her we are becoming her.

And the exciting part is that we never complete the journey. Just when we think we have hit our stride and we are indeed a shining example of a fiery and fabulous women in her third act, and that our lives couldn't get any better… BAM! We hit the next level of richness in our lives and we start again from this new stage. As the universe continues to expand we, too, expand with her.

A self-empowered life
When we really get rolling forward living from this new place of freedom that comes to us in our third act it seems to take on a life of its own. Our new way of living and taking full responsibility for our health and happiness is in our hands and we are now gliding on the energy of a self-empowered life. No one is going to live our life for us and we wouldn't want them to. As a matter of fact, fiery, fabulous women won't let anyone live their life for them! So, sacred sisters, let's get to it!

All of your choices—good and not so good—were your choices and they served you in some way at the time, so be proud of how you have lived your life and the things you chose to give your time and attention too. I know that because you are reading this book you are past choosing things for yourself that don't increase your life force. So, tossing out the vile jar of slime will be an easy choice to make.

Keep the wisdom, toss the judgement.

You are now creating space for yourself to breathe and move and enjoy your life and to fully get to know yourself again. I am finding that for myself it has been like meeting someone for the first time that seems very familiar to me, a bit of a *déjà vue* experience. Even though I can feel my new self is alive and thriving I also still feel that part of me that has a heart of fire, the wild part of me that continues to burn with passion for life and it made me think about that term "young at heart". In my 30's and 40's that applied to me for sure and, as much as I thought it still did, it actually doesn't. I'm on to the next stage and young at heart is too lightweight for me now.

As the years go by and more of the wisdom I now walk with reveals itself, a more fitting thing to say about myself and women thriving in their third act is, "hearts on fire". There are many things that catch the eye and the interest of women over fifty. We are making it a priority to let the things that we are passionate about be the things that turn our smouldering embers into flames. We are no longer "young at heart" but women with hearts on fire. Which may explain those hot flashes!

Let's get into creative play mode now and start the Know Yourself process by playing the lottery game. Perhaps you have played this before, it's called, **"Everything I would do**

if I won the lottery."

If this is your first time playing, I welcome you to the fun! Now go ahead and take a few breaths and start to imagine yourself as the lottery winner and for the sake of some semblance of rules to this game let's all play as if we won the same amount say, **Sixty Million Dollars**. This was inspired by the amount of a big lottery draw that happened last night. Let's go with this amount since it is real to someone out there today.

Begin with how you feel as you look at your ticket and the moment you realize the sixty million is yours. See yourself at the lottery office receiving your cheque. Now see your bank account with sixty million dollars in it. Yes, it is perfectly alright to have a huge smile on your face right now. We *are* practicing feeling like we have won the lottery. Smiling would most certainly show up in the handbook on, "*What to do when you win the lottery.*"

Go ahead and let a big-ass grin take over your whole face right now. Heck, you can even yell out, "I won!"

Get into it, ladies. It is our game, our imagination, and we can get as far into it as we are willing to let ourselves go.

Now begin to feel how your heart and mind accept that you are able to do any and all things that make your heart sing. Feel it and trust it as truth. Begin now to play-plan the way you will spend your money. This is the fun part because with sixty million dollars you can do anything in your wildest dreams. You can just put the book down for 5–10 minutes now and dream away.

Welcome back from your imaginative journey of absolute freedom. Did you spend all of your money? Did you give it all away to your favorite people and places? Did you really get into it? Did you see yourself having a great time? Did you get into humanitarian projects bringing fresh drinking water and education to communities without these things in place? Did you hire someone to drive you around everywhere you wanted to go? How far did you go into imagining yourself swimming in the absolute freedom sixty million dollars could bring you?

Did you find that you began to create limitations where there were none? Did you start to think about who you wouldn't share with? Did you take more time planning how you would save, invest and hoard your winnings than choosing all of the things that would increase your health and happiness?

How we respond to a game that lets us play with the idea of absolute freedom, and what we would do with that freedom, gives us a good indication of how much freedom we believe we are allowed to enjoy. As well it's a great indication of what actually does bring us joy.

What was the first thing you thought of? To take a luxury trip to a destination you have dreamed of? Well now you know you walk with the spark of travel in your heart. So, write in your journal or in the margin here "I love to travel."

Who did you bring with you? Write the names of those people down, too, because they are the ones you desire to share your time with. The next time you are making your way (traveling) to visit a person or a place you have never been before, think about how much you love to travel, and that you have an adventurous spirit even if you are simply taking the bus to a new part of the city. We can start to see that our lives are filled with more every day adventure when we open our minds up to unlimited thinking.

Did you hire a personal chef with your winnings? I always do! So, in my journal it says, "I love eating well!"

You can go ahead and make a few notes also of the places you held yourself back. Did you run out of creative ways to spend your sixty million dollars? Did you spend more time plotting how you would get someone else to collect the winnings for you so certain people in your life would never find out you were crazy rich? Write their names down, too. These folks are likely the ones who will challenge your growth process.

If intuitively you know that you need to hide your good fortune from someone in your life then you will eventually need to look at rebranding, restructuring or releasing those relationships. We can do that directly with the person or we can do it without them if we shift the way we perceive people and the way we react to our more challenging relationships. Many times it is enough to shift the whole relationship into something beneficial for everyone. Remember we are taking responsibility for our happiness and ninety percent of our happiness comes by choosing it.

This is all just information, we are trying to get to know ourselves more intimately and this is all part of the unearthing of our current state of being. Our hearts and minds are full of rich and interesting information. For many of us this will be the first time we were able to see that we have been holding ourselves back and keeping our imaginations small. I play this game quite often.

Go ahead and chose on a scale of 1-10: How free did you feel during the Know Yourself exercise? 1 being not very free at all, but more stuck and 10 being so free to enjoy the game that you could have happily played on.

Circle your position on our scale now.

1   2   3   4   5   6   7   8   9   10

Add this game to your practice, play it occasionally or often as you want, and begin to observe where you are in your life and how that effects the freedom of your imagination and your ability to see yourself completely free from worry and complaints.

Harvard's Grant Glueck Study of Happiness

Activist Melanie Curtin wrote a fantastic piece where she gives us a clear picture of the results of the *Harvard Happiness Study*, conducted over a 75-year period. I highly recommend reading her full article (link is in the Resources section), but I will give you a few of the highlights from it here to whet your happiness whistle.

Robert Waldinger, director of the Harvard Study of Adult Development says, "The clearest message that we get from this 75-year study is this: Good relationships keep us happier and healthier. Period. It's not just the number of friends you have, and it's not whether or not you're in a committed relationship. It's the quality of your close relationships that matters."

The Pursuit of Happiness

Imagine if you will, that we are in the pursuit of happiness together. That you understand and truly feel that what we are doing is, instead of moving forward like explorers of land and sea, we are diving inside of ourselves, deep into the well of happiness that is within us. Our practices are our physical, emotional and spiritual road to travel. We are walking inward towards the layers of happiness, fulfillment and understanding that we have been cultivating for over fifty years. We have a foundation of wisdom within us, a foundation of street smarts that is acquired solely due to the number of days we have lived.

We have a foundation of happiness within us that we are stepping up onto like a stepping on the stage of our life well-lived. As we continue breathing with focus each day, we will be taken deeper into ourselves. The journey is inward and often confusing because we have been programed to look outside of ourselves for most things in this life.

I want to honour that part of our journey also, that accumulation part of our journey where we have collected houses and cars and furniture, as well as letters after our names, awards and respect for our work of raising families and raising ourselves into an incredible expression of who we are. Now we stand strong on all of those foundations and we breathe.

I'm not trying to tell you how to do it, I'm only saying put some pride into it. Be what you are my friend and live the life.
— The Staples Singers
"Be What You Are"

Then what happens is that we become calmer. More at ease with ourselves. We become interested in ourselves, not simply just more accepting of our current state, but truly interested in all of the experiences that got us to this point and interested in where we may go from here. We become well practiced in being in the present moment.

Take a Magical Moment breath right here, right now. The only thing you need to bring focus to is:

Inhale, retain, exhale, pause...

Inhale, retain, exhale, pause...

Inhale, retain, exhale, pause...

That is the Magical Moment breath we give ourselves every day. Choose when you can fit it in and do it.

Our Third Sacred Practice

Our Daily Statement

Today I open myself fully to living a sacred life, I call in now the people, places and things that lift me up, light me up and hold me up as the accountable, responsible and authentic woman I am here to be. And so it is.

The Know Yourself Imagination Practice (Imagining/Thoughts)

Your imagination practice is the game "Everything I would I do if I Won the Lottery." (NOTE: This is a condensed version of the game you just played above.)

How fun! A creative game of liberating your mind and heart from restraints and old programs.

Play as often as you like and keep an eye on how your scale of 1-10 shifts when there are changes in your life and your attitude.

This is not only a fun practice, it is also very serious to me. I use a similar one in my meditation groups. It is serious to me because of its ability to expose the truth of where we are mentally as well as emotionally in our lives. It can show us where we are around trust and help to free us from living programs that belong to other people, or that are now outdated for us.

Imagine now that you are checking your lottery ticket and you realize you have won.

Feel winning flood over your body.

Now go ahead and take a few breaths and start to imagine yourself as the lottery winner and of **Sixty Million Dollars**.

Begin with how you feel as you look at your ticket and the moment you realize the sixty million is yours. See yourself at the lottery office receiving your cheque. Now see your bank account with sixty million dollars in it. Yes, it is perfectly alright to have a huge smile on your face right now. We *are* practicing feeling like we have won the lottery. Smiling would most certainly show up in the handbook on, "*What to do when you win the lottery.*"

Go ahead and let a big grin take over your whole face right now. You can even yell out, "I won!"

Get into it. Ladies. It is our game, our imagination, and we can get as far into it as we are willing to let ourselves go.

Now begin to feel how your heart and mind accept that you can do any, and all of the things that make your heart sing.

Feel it and trust it as truth.

Begin now to play-plan the way you will spend your

money. This is the fun part because with sixty million dollars you can do anything in your wildest dreams. You can just put the book down for 5–10 minutes now and dream away.

Go ahead and chose, on a scale of 1–10, how **free** did you feel during the Know Yourself imagination exercise? 1 being not very free at all, but more stuck

10 being so free to enjoy the game that you could have happily played on.

Circle your position on our scale now.

1   2   3   4   5   6   7   8   9   10

Keep doing a check in with your scale of 1-10 on how free you feel doing this exercise, until you feel so free that spending sixty million dollars is a piece of cake to you!

If I could get my point across in this book in two words and an exclamation mark it would be. Have Fun!

Because this is the point now.

**The Know Yourself Breathing Practice
(Breathing/Words)**
Do this exercise from a seated position.

Inhale, retain, exhale, and pause.

Continue to breathe from the four parts of your breath.

Now we use a simple variation of alternate nostril breathing to balance our mind and bodies as we become more acquainted with ourselves and how it feels to be more relaxed and live from a deeper place of calm.

Take your thumb, using the tip of your thumb to cover your right nostril so you block air from entering this side.

Inhale deeply on your left side, then retain your breath.

While you retain your breath switch your thumb to your left nostril.

Now exhale out of the right nostril.

Pause.

Keep the left side covered, inhale deeply on your right side.

Retain your breath.

Switch and cover your right-side nostril.

Exhale deeply on the left.

Inhale left side.

Retain your breath and switch.

Cover left and exhale right side.

Keep this going, switching back and forth, slow and steady for a full minute.

Pause, then do another round if you'd like.

Really enjoy the pause after this practice, luxuriate in your breathing and in the space once you have completed the practice.

The Know Yourself Physical Practice (Physical/Actions)

This is a balance posture to get to know ourselves. A physical balance practice also helps us to understand the levels of balance in our lives emotionally, and mentally. Take your time, use a counter or a weighted piece of furniture to hold on to on days you need help with balance.

Level One: Begin by gently rolling through your feet a time or two, putting all your weight into the toes then the heels, toes then the heels. Begin to feel grounded in both feet equally.

Now shift your weight side to side, all your weight to the right foot so the left foot feels slightly lifted.

Shift all your weight into the left foot with the right foot feeling slightly lifted.

You can do this for a few breaths, even up to a full minute.

Tip: Bend your knees slightly as you do this, you are in a flow. Do not lock your knees. That is too stiff for what we are going for here.

Continue side to side and when you feel that you're balanced and connected well into your feet and the flow, begin to raise one knee up.

Shift and raise the other knee up.

Gently moving with your breath, side to side

Bring the knees up as high or as low as you prefer.

Level Two: Tree pose. A traditional yoga posture for balance, strength, and self-reflection.

Shift all your weight into your right foot and bring your left foot off the ground.

You have a couple of options:

You can keep your left toes on the floor and simply put your heel to your ankle;

Or you can lift your foot up and place it between your ankle and your knee;

Or you can bring your foot right up between your knee and your hip, you'll need use your hand to help lift your foot into position.

You may want to use the wall, a table or a solid chair to help you learn to maintain your balance.

Your hands are at your heart in prayer position, palms together at the heart. Breathe deeply and balance. If you like, raise your arms up over head and wide.

You could take them low and wide if you have any tension in your shoulders, or any variation you like. Try many!

Hold for as long as you can do it comfortably then gently switch sides, and repeat. Your breath is a smooth and even, inhale, retain, exhale, and pause.

In balance postures we're not only cultivating physical balance but emotional and mental balance too. Observe your thoughts while you balance, especially on the days when you're falling out of your posture. See if you can find humour in that, instead of judgment. Slow and steady, one day at a time, cultivating balance in mind, body, and spirit and really getting to know yourself.

Chapter Four

THE FOURTH SACRED RESPONSIBILITY: COLLABORATE

I can promise you that women working together—linked, informed and educated—can bring peace and prosperity to this forsaken planet.

—Isabel Allende

Having help, getting help, asking for help, and accepting help are all the empowering practices of someone who knows Collaboration as a Sacred Responsibility. There are three aspects to collaboration I have observed so far.

First there is the collaboration that happens when we consciously step into the role of Collaborator, to help or serve another.

Second when we accept or encourage another to work with us or help us.

The third collaboration reveals itself in the natural world, like the collaboration between the moon and the tides, the between seed and soil, and between the trillions of cells in our bodies working together so that we may thrive. Over 35 trillion cells in our body, and one of the greatest examples of collaboration of all times!

There is collaboration everywhere and we need it to survive as well as thrive. We are a collaboration of fiery and fabulous women walking a sacred path together, each one of us contributing to the universal collaboration in our authentic and unique way.

Sacred Reciprocity: a fancy term for collaboration

I call the great collaboration in the cycles of giving and receiving Sacred Reciprocity. This Sacred Reciprocity is found in our breath. On the inhale we receive, on the exhale we give. It can be found during our exchanges in conversations where we find the best conversations have an uplifting quality that comes from a balance of listening and speaking. We find Sacred Reciprocity in our relationships where all people are respected and the exchange of loving duties to the relationships are shared equally.

Sacred Reciprocity does not mean a 50/50 equal split on everything although it does ride the middle path in that way. As we are needed to support each other we will find that sometimes we are giving more and receiving less, and sometimes we receive more and give less. There is an ebb and flow as we move through life, give support and receive support.

It is crucial for our energy levels to be well maintained and that we keep Sacred Reciprocity at the front of our hearts and minds. As you have begun cultivating your Self-Care practices, you will be better able to see the dance and the balance of sacred reciprocity in your lives and use your observations to serve your own energy levels with respect.

We are now experimenting with keeping our energy

at the healthiest levels possible and this is dependent on how balanced the energy in and energy out is in our lives. When we find that people, places or things increase our vitality, being in those situations is like filling up our energy bank account, it is a collaboration of energies swimming in sacred reciprocity. We now go to the places, and do the things, with the most supportive people that increase our energy levels because we understand that it is our level of energy propelling us forward or holding us back.

Together we are stronger
It is not a symbol of strength to avoid asking for support or to work together and saying you don't want to bother anyone, or you don't need anyone's help, you are just fine on your own, if you want it done right you might as well do it yourself or any other BS excuse you tell yourself not to trust and enjoy collaboration.

We simply do not survive without each other and we most certainly do not thrive as a species alone. Both our health and happiness are compromised when we lack community and connection. All things in nature are in an integrated cycle and we know that we are not separate from nature. We are set up, or hardwired if you will, for connection.

On a recent radio program, they were discussing how more and more people are dying from loneliness. Just let that land for a moment. What is going on in a world populated with billions of people and we are dying of loneliness? When I heard this news, I felt heartbroken and I began to wonder how this could be—and frankly I began to watch my own behavior more closely.

Was I the best neighbor I could be? Did I spend the time to hear the older lady from the fifth floor of my building to tell me her snippets of news gathered from her morning walk? I wanted to know if I actually left people feeling like a caring connection had been made when we crossed paths.

Did I hold a door, or take a caring pause, and actually look someone in the eye when I said hello as we passed in the hallway? Was I too busy, or too late, or too darn important for someone? Were my grocery bags too heavy to stand and listen to someone for a few moments? Was the weight of my apples and carrots more important than a human interaction?

I began to observe myself and I found I had an opportunity to change a little. To slow down a little. What I discovered is that I was a pretty good neighbor. But to be a great neighbor I was going to have to up my game! So, I began to leave my apartment a bit earlier than necessary so that if I ran into someone on my way to the car I could relax and enjoy an extended hello or listen to a story or two from one of the older folks in the building.

To be perfectly honest, I have no idea if my self-inquiry is helping anyone feel any less lonely, but I don't need to have an end game or an equal exchange here. I don't need to know anything other than I took a piece of information that affected my heart and I found a way to accept responsibility in a way that made sense to me and in a way that I could truly act as a change-maker in my own life.

It is our mistake to believe we can't make a difference unless we are part of a more elaborate activity like a march, a rally, or a protest. Ladies attend them, attend them in great numbers, but also join forces close to home.

In the beginning, there was collaboration

From conception to exiting this life, we make connections with one and other. Let's take it from the top and look at pre-conception, as a couple makes the decision to collaborate on bringing a child into the world, then the reciprocal relationship between mother and growing baby. Between the expectant parents during pregnancy. There is collaboration in raising the child not only from the parents but from the extended family of grandparents, aunties, uncles, brothers and sisters. It extends out into the community as friends and neighbors all contribute to the wellbeing of our families. Straight up, it takes a village to raise a child and it takes collaboration.

As we begin to really understand that collaboration is everywhere and integral for us to thrive, we can start viewing the world from this perspective. From this viewpoint we now act and live as if everyone is on our team, and we feel it. Feeling it is key to thriving in our connections and it is the part we have to practice most, to truly feel ourselves as part of a whole. Part of the wholeness of life. This is the part where we start to understand in our hearts and minds that indeed we are part of something greater than simply our individual journey. That is highly respected also, but now we have an expanded understanding of our contribution to the greater collaboration of life.

Collaborating in relationships as a sacred woman

We are on a journey of Self-Care, Knowing our Self, Self-Inquiry and Self-Discovery. That is a whole lot of focus on our self, and none of it is selfish until we stop collaborating with others. It is a fine art to shift into our third act and support everyone around us during our own process of renewal and, dare I say it, the thing we all resist most, change. And, as if it is not hard enough coming to terms with our own change we need to manage the changes in those who are closest to us, too.

If we position ourselves to be on top of, or above others we will inevitably exhaust ourselves building that platform alone. Yes, we want to continually elevate in our levels of joy, gratitude, and creativity but we take others with us through inspiration, cooperation and collaboration. You will be at the top of your game, this I can assure you, and you will have arrived there by way of your practices, and celebration of all who collaborated with you on your journey. You will not have gotten to the top of your game without the collaboration of like hearted people who stood beside you, who related to you at pivotal times, who celebrated, loved, and believed in you.

We also give great thanks to the ones who didn't stand beside us when we needed them. The one person we held closest to us we thought failed us when we needed the most intimacy and support. The ones we needed to be more courageous than we were able to be at a particular time in our lives. It is here that these people from my life are honoured. As you read it, feel it apply to you and those in your life with whom you have a similar experience.

Thank you to those who have distracted me, pulled me off course, put me down, and tried to dim my light. I have learned so much from each of you about self-respect, keeping myself safe, and raising myself up at my lowest points.

You have all been a sacred gift to my resilience. I am grateful for your short, but lesson-filled, time in my life. May your journey be blessed.

These people are a rich part of our life's tapestry and the sooner we release our disappointment in them or ourselves for choosing those relationships in the first place the sooner we can thrive in the wisdom that came from our experiences with them. Many times, those are the exact relationships that make us fight for our own happiness, respect and freedom to thrive joyously in our lives.

The next time you find yourself talking or thinking about those who disappointed you or judging yourself for letting those people close to you, flip the script and take sacred responsibility for your happiness.

Write down one thing (or many) that you learned from that particular relationship. If you are not able to write when those thoughts surface, then take your three Magical Moment breaths and allow one thing you can identify as wisdom to come into your mind. Sometimes the wisdom is, "I now know how I don't want to be treated."

Whatever the wisdom is in that moment, name it, then send it from your mind to your heart. Let the wisdom leave an imprint on your heart and set free the disappointment you have been hosting in your mind, if only for a moment. Do this as often as the need arises. This is a collaboration of the heart and mind for your freedom from attachment and, therefore, suffering.

This is an ongoing practice and, believe me, finding the wisdom in our places of pain can be like finding a needle in a haystack most times. But what we have now, ladies, is the power of being in our third act. There is something special that moves into us at this time of our lives, a new level of strength, a more flexible foundation. Perhaps it is the desire to enjoy our lives more fully than ever before, or it is the maturity of our minds or the wild fire burning in our hearts that seem to 'burn off' the burden of carrying disappointment. Whatever it is, it is in service to us now and we will receive it with open arms. Bring on forgiveness! Bring on letting go of all the things that no longer serve our greater good! Bring on collaboration with freedom!

Life Cycles and Collaboration

Consider the ways you see cycles unfolding in your life. Understand in your bones that all things have a cycle. The cycle that takes us from one day to the next, morning, noon, night and the dreamtime. The human cycle of birth and death each one of us is on the path of right now. The birth and death cycles of plants and animals. The cycles of the seasons throughout the year.

Really begin to see all the places our lives are informed by cycles as part of your natural day to day observance. Acknowledging these cycles we all live with is a powerful way of deepening our appreciation for our own lives as well as our connection to the natural world. Start to see the cycles in everything around you and honour that everything has both a beginning and end as well as a rich space of experiences that goes on between the two, including the journey of your own life.

Having conversations about the cycle of birth and death for most of us is often like someone tossed a hot potato into the room, but it is a fascinating topic regarding knowing ourselves. For just a moment, take a few breaths and think about your response to the cycle of birth and death. What comes to your mind as you sit considering the flow of the cycles in your life and the lives of others close to you.

How comfortable are you discussing life and death? How frank and relaxed are you when you find yourself in a conversation about death? How responsible would you say you are around your own after-life arrangements? Will you donate your beautiful organs when you pass? Have you talked with loved ones about your wishes when your life is complete? As the wise women in our circles, it will most likely be us taking the lead in conversations like this and mentoring others on the natural cycles of life and the plain old facts of being in these fabulous human bodies.

On a scale of 1-10 circle how comfortable are you with the conversation of death with #1 being "I can't bear to think about it" and #10 being "I feel fully at peace with this part of the life cycle."

1	2	3	4	5	6	7	8	9	10

There is no right or wrong answer, just simply identifying where we are at this particular moment in connection and collaboration with the natural cycles of life.

My dear teacher and mentor of Toltec wisdom, HeatherAsh Amara speaks to this in her book, *Warrior Goddess Training: Becoming the Woman You Are Meant to Be*. In her section on Cyclical Living she says it beautifully.

When we align with life, we choose to align with all of life, not just the parts we like or are comfortable with—and not just when everything goes our way. Aligning with life means truly knowing and accepting that aging, death, sickness, natural disasters, accidents, humans and their wacky ways—all these things are bound to alter our course. Aligning with life means understanding that you cannot control the cycles of nature.

Links to HeatherAsh Amara's website and contact info are in the resources section. All of her books are considered recommended reading for fiery and fabulous women!

Know that you are supported by the flow of foundational living. This is where we build foundations in the areas of our lives that most support our vitality and our ability to thrive. Continue building foundations in your relationships as this is our cornerstone of collaboration as a sacred responsibility. Allow yourself to build a strong foundation of understanding on how you relate to this world and its cycles and let it be a guiding light.

The women I love and admire for their strength and grace did not get that way because shit worked out. They got that way because shit went wrong, and they handled it. They handled it a thousand different ways on a thousand different days, but they handled it. Those women are my superheroes.
—Elizabeth Gilbert.

Collaboration also touches the we-are-one perspective. We are all connected, yes, we are individuals, yes, but we are each a thread on the grand tapestry of life. Allow your thread to be strong, pliable and resilient. In a world of collaboration, we can liberate ourselves from separation consciousness, loneliness, and isolation as we trust ourselves to work together lovingly in deep relationship to everything that is conspiring to support us. The quality of our life is directly related to the quality of our relationships and collaboration is the key.

Our Fourth Sacred Practice

Our Daily Statement

Today I open myself fully to living a sacred life, I call in now the people, places and things that lift me up, light me up and hold me up as the accountable, responsible and authentic woman I am here to be. And so it is.

The Collaborate Imagination Practice (Imagining/Thoughts)

Today we are cultivating a daily practice of non-harming as we honour the Sacred Responsibility of Collaboration. We have a day where there is nothing we do that harms another being, including ourselves of course. Our thoughts, words, and actions are in harmony with collaboration and *Ahimsa* the yogic principal of non-harming.

This exercise begins with our imagination setting the stage and we carry it out into our physical day. A collaboration of imagination and present moment action.

Imagine now that you are observing yourself go about your day as you normally would.

Imagine you are observing a day in your own life from a few feet above your body.

Imagine you are out of your body and in your sweet soul, hovering gently over you, observing and guiding you, as you move through your day of non-harming.

Imagine observing yourself wake up and stretch and then make your way to wash your face and brush your teeth.

Imagine observing your interaction with yourself in the mirror, how you interact with the water and imagine yourself in such gratitude for all that you have in this moment.

Imagine yourself going about your day, interacting with people, animals, plants and the elements, all from a place of non-harming.

Imagine a full day of non-harming from the time you wake up to the time you lay your head down on your pillow. Just walk yourself through an imaginary day of non-harming as you go.

Take as long as you like to visualize that everywhere you go and everything you do is coming from a place of ease, peace, joy, and no harm.

Like all of our imagination practices, they are never over when we think we are finished. This is part of the brilliance of imagining and visualizing, it is like dropping a pebble in a pond, these practices continue to ripple out into our day. You will find yourself connecting with non-harming as you make choices, observe your thoughts, words, and actions and even those of others you interact with. Hold your ground on your practice of non-harming.

If you find yourself up against a situation where you are unsure of how to respond, ask yourself the three questions of a conscious, caring person.

Will this harm me?

Will this harm someone else?

Will this harm my environment?

Observe how deeply you can celebrate your day of non-harming. Have reverence for all of the living things around you and keeping your connection to the natural world in the forefront of this practice.

It relaxes the nervous system to be kind, and it will agitate the nervous system to act in ways that are unkind, and agitation is for washing machines, not our hearts.

The Collaborate Breathing Practice (Breathing/Words)

Our breathing practice is a collaboration between breath and imagination.

Begin to settle into your natural breathing pattern of inhale, retain, exhale, and pause.

Get centred in your body, bringing your awareness to the physical centre of your body, wherever that is for you. Maybe it's your heart centre, maybe the solar plexus, maybe low in your belly. Find the space that feels like centre for you today.

Imagine that you are being mentored on collaboration by the cycles of the day.

See yourself waking up as the sun begins to rise.

Begin to imagine now that you are in collaboration with everyone and everything in your life.

Imagine yourself as you prepare your first meal of the day.

Imagine how all the ingredients collaborate to create an incredible taste experience.

Imagine now how the beautiful fresh water you have filled the kettle with is in collaboration with the bubbles dancing within as your tea water boils.

Imagine your gratitude for the collaboration between boiling water and kettle.

Continue to imagine collaboration between the hot water and the tea leaves you are steeping.

Looking deeper at the collaboration of mixed plants that created your morning tea.

The collaboration between cup and handle, handle and hand, hand and fingers.

Begin to deeply experience collaboration and the gratitude that comes when you experience all of the things that support you on your journey of collaboration.

Continue to imagine all the ways you are supported by the nature of collaboration in your day.

Imagine yourself walking out of your home and responding to the collaboration between feet and the ground as you walk, feet connecting, ground supporting.

Notice the collaboration between foot and shoe, between shoe and laces, and so on.

In a practice of observing collaboration from the tiniest of possibilities to the largest possibilities we begin to increase our levels of rich appreciation for all of the many ways we are supported by a symphony of collaboration. Even honouring each muscle in our face collaborating to produce our beautiful smile.

Allow your imagination practice to come and go in your mind naturally throughout your day. Continuing to observe collaboration all around you, finding yourself in a collaborative flow where there is space for everyone and everything to support each other. As we keep an open-hearted connection to collaboration it becomes nearly impossible to see ourselves as separate from the natural world or alone in this world.

The Collaborate Physical Practice (Physical/Actions)

This exercise is a collaboration of flow, strength, balance, movement, and breath. This exercise is meant to be done standing yet can be done in a seated position by simply engaging in the upper body portion of the exercise.

Stand with your feet comfortably wide apart, much wider than hip width while maintaining stability for this practice.

Toes slightly turned out, your knees and toes will go in the same direction.

Now go ahead and drop into your seat. As if you were sitting on an invisible chair.

Knees bend as little or as much as is comfortable for this wide leg squat.

As you get stronger you can squat deeper.

Take your hands to your heart in prayer position.

Breathe deeply and feel the strength in your body starting with the connection of your feet to the earth.

Stay in this position for a few breaths.

Beginning your collaboration with balance, focus, and strength.

Taking a deep breath now, inhale.

As you exhale your right hand will cross your body pressing your palm towards the left.

Inhale bring your hand back to prayer position at your heart.

Exhale left hand crosses your body pressing your palm towards the right.

Inhale bring your left hand back to your heart.

Exhale and reach your right hand across your body pressing as far as you can go.

Inhale right hand comes back to prayer position.

Exhale left hand crosses the body pressing far as you can go.

Matching your breath and your movement as a collaboration.

Continue and do as many as you're comfortable with, eventually working yourself up to three sets of eight, or as many as you love.

Chapter Five

The Fifth Sacred Responsibility: Honour your Intuition

A strong woman understands that the gifts such as logic, decisiveness, and strength are just as feminine as intuition and emotional connection. She values and uses all of her gifts.

—*Nancy Rathburn*

For goodness sake, rip the Band-Aid off, ladies! It is time to honour our intuition for the incredible inner compass that it is. Call it what you will but we have a keen inner knowing that can be continuously traced back to the start of something that was fabulous for us, *and* the start of something that totally sucked. I have ignored my intuition many times in my life and doing that set me back a few steps each time. But at this stage of my game I find it exhilarating to follow my intuition! Intuition can be extremely subtle as well as it can blast your heart or mind wide open.

Everything you need you already have inside of you. Signals, feelings, knowing's and inner voice are all aspects of intuition and taking Sacred Responsibility for Honouring your Intuition is your brilliant roadmap to your life well lived.

Respecting the inner wisdom keeper

When experiencing an emotional expression of intuition, we can feel our own intuition or even someone else's feelings. It is essential to respect our own inner wisdom keeper as well as another's inner knowing. It is our sacred responsibility never to block someone else's intuition from being expressed. When someone tells you something doesn't feel right, they are actually trusting you with their vulnerability. It is a vulnerable act of courage when we listen to and act from our intuitive sense. As a woman who takes sacred responsibility to honour her intuition she also models that to others. And, when trusted with someone's vulnerable sharing of their intuitive sense we receive that as a sacred responsibility to be loyal not only to the person trusting us enough to share, but also our loyalty to the sacredness of the intuitive knowing of all of us. We stand with each other empowered by the gift of human intuition.

The Intellect, Data and Intuition

Understand this, ladies, we don't just sit around and wonder if we are "tuned into" our intuition. We don't wait for our intuition to reveal itself to us. We gently and regularly cultivate our connection to the way we feel intuitive messages in our bodies. The same way we develop our muscles, we develop our intuition. I would love to issue a blanket statement that, "intuition is a natural part of the human experience" and that is very true, but so is being physically strong and emotionally balanced. Yet we still must put effort into keeping these things in fine form.

When intellect and intuition intersect we find ourselves in places of curiosity, questioning, and learning. We build up our data banks of understanding and experiences through our own lives and the lives of others who mentor us. We listen to each other's life stories, we do research, we read, observe, and we lean into our lives. All the information we actively collect by living our lives as interested and interesting women is part of creating our own personal data base from which to pull. The more we data we have in our personal data banks, the easier it is to distinguish between our reactions to things (like our idea of how things "should be" or our judgements about things we don't understand) and our actual intuitive sense.

Our intellectual interests in life are a big part of cultivating our connection to our intuition. We can watch documentaries, read great books, visit new places, learn about different cultures, and look up random subjects on the internet once in a while. We become open to all the many ways we can enjoy new and interesting information for our data base.

In this way of digging into life, we become more well-rounded in our approach to life, more accepting, and our lack of understanding others no longer clouds us. All of this allows our intuitive sense to sharpen and guide us.

The Voice of Intuition
Intuition speaks like the blink of lighthouse, a flash of insight. The message is brief, clear, and registers in the body

and mind at once, "go" or "don't go". Its sleight of hand essence makes it easy to ignore especially when we are not fully present in the moment. Because the intuitive message touches both our body and mind it resonates strongly. We typically describe intuition as a "gut feeling". A message may seem to come and go, but if it is an intuitive message we find it still sitting in our gut.

Intuition can be a part of a general good or bad feeling we have about something. But, beware! The quick voice of intuition can get drowned out by louder voices coming from the mental mind. A clue we are in the mental mind is if there is a lot of uncertainty going on in our head around an issue. "Should I go, I should, it will look good if I do, and mom will be happy if I do it because she was last time."

This kind of mental chatter is the mind distracting us from intuition and presenting us with the evidence of our stored data. While our evidence can be convincing, sometimes it is distorted by a "nervous ego" which will be working hard at putting forward all the evidence it can so that it can stay alive in its opinion. Good evidence is made of wisdom and true knowledge, yet the difficulty is that we often can't discern the difference between ego evidence and true knowledge.

Intuition is a unique guidance system. It is a flash of information that resonates in the body. Go. Don't go. You feel it. You got it. And you know that not listening and acting in your best and sacred interest will bring an outcome with, let's say… "lots of learning opportunity."

Intuition and Intimate Relationships

Our intimate relationships are the most amazing places to honour our intuition. In our intimate relationships, we have the blessing of being the closest we can be with another person. We get to be 100% our authentic selves, allowing us a safe place to experiment with our own intimate life experiences and our intuitive senses.

Recently, I was catching up with a good friend and it included a bit of a check-in on where I was at since the recent parting of ways with the "man of my dreams". As we dissected the bitter truths about how he and I jumped from a place of happily-ever-after to heartbreak overnight, she asked me a simple question, "Did you see any red flags at the beginning?"

Well, there you have it. When her question reached my ears I just knew, in all of my cells, I knew. Yes, I did see red flags. Actually, I heard red flags, and that was even worse for me to reconcile.

It was in that moment that I had to face the sobering fact that I had abandoned my intuition in some spiritual attempt to accept someone fully because that is what a kind, spiritual person would do, right? I was protecting someone else's hurtful behaviour in the name of some overt kindness that actually didn't include being kind to me.

I gotta tell you, sisters, I am so over ignoring my intuition. If you feel something is "off" in the relationship, chances are it is. *That* is your intuition talking.

When we ignore those intuitive pangs that something is out of alignment for us, we actual do a disservice to the other person and the relationship as a whole. If we ignore our intuition in our intimate relationships we will give our partner a false sense that there are no concerns, and that is unfair to them, to you, and all of the family and friends who support your relationship together.

Sometimes we just love someone so much that we can't bear to tell them we are not in alignment with their words or actions. But love yourself equally and be brave. People are amazing and most times they will surprise you and love you up. They will be grateful that you trusted them so much that you shared your sense something was off.

As sovereign sacred women, we are the ones who will likely take the lead in the open-hearted conversations when our intuitive sense has risen to the surface in our most intimate relationships. Even when feeling hurt, we discern the information from our data banks and we communicate from an empowered place of vulnerable knowing, and we always communicate with love because that's how we roll!

Treat Yourself Like Someone You Love

I take responsibility for my past choices of ignoring my intuition, my instinctive knowing, my gut, and those red flags. I take full responsibility and I will pass on the wisdom that came from doing that.

There is nothing more spiritual than accepting others exactly as they choose to be, and in that philosophy being true to your own happiness. Go ahead and make the space between you and someone treating you in ways out of sync with your intuitive senses. But while you make that space please continue to advocate for kindness and growth in your relationships and use your skills of sacred responsibility when your intuitive sense tells you something doesn't feel right.

Learn the difference between a real intuitive sense in your body, and your mind trying to make sense of something you are unsure of, or cannot relate to, and do it from a place of non-attachment and as an observer.

Choosing to spend less time with people who don't lift you up is perfectly fine. You may need to release some people from your life altogether if they are abusive. That is not only perfectly fine, it is our sacred responsibility to have people in our lives who respect our hearts. Either find ways to grow in kindness together or create a wide berth.

The truth is, your life is made up of your own choices, follow your intuition, choose respect, choose kindness and always choose compassion.

Beware of the Change-back Monster

For those of you hearing about the Change-back Monster for the first time, welcome to the reality that when we change someone will inevitably want to point it out as a bad thing, something wrong, or even laugh at us and our efforts to change.

We are social creatures and our social system is designed to stay the way it is. Whenever you try to make changes in your life there are going to be people around you who are either consciously or unconsciously threatened by the "new you."

Change-back Monsters come in all forms with all the tricks and angles to get us to "change back" to the exact way they are comfortable with us being. And when we were

Any person who undergoes a dramatic shift creates a ripple effect, requiring change from others around her/him. So they will work again either consciously or unconsciously to sabotage your efforts getting you to Change-back to the same old you that they are comfortable with.

—Martha Beck

younger and less determined to take sacred responsibility for our happiness they may have been able to pull us back into their comfort zone.

My dear friend, and the editor of this book, Kirsten, and I created a workbook-supported program called *Making Wealthy Choices* and right in the middle of the program we address the Change-back Monster in detail. I share some of it here so that we can continue to rise up and not be held back by people who, for the most part, just need to know that they are safe and loved even when you change. Change-back Monsters can have a detrimental effect on how we trust our intuition, as they can be very convincing, mostly because we love the "old us" too. But now in our third act, we are changing things up!

My Mini Monster Example

One Saturday night I got an email from a friend who asked me how my day had been. I sent back an enthusiastic message about how I had spent the whole afternoon and into the evening writing and recording content for the programs and I was thrilled with everything.

The response I got was, "That's all fine and good Cath, but there is a whole world out there to explore, do you think you are going to leave your apartment tomorrow and get some fresh air?"

Now *that* was a sneak attack on the positive changes that I was making in my life. And what do you think happened when I read that email? Yeah, that's right. Someone burst my bubble. And for a millisecond I doubted the use of my time.

Oh, I wanted to send back a big email back, defending my use of time, and how what I was doing was going to help so many people, instead I only wrote one line.

"Have you ever heard of the Change-back Monster?"

And actually, what I experienced was pretty mild; the most surprising Change-back attacks come from those who are closest to us—intimate partners and family members. And it can sting when our closest people don't celebrate our change right out of the gate.

Mostly, people mean well but that doesn't mean we have to change back. But it does mean that we don't get an automatic pass to joy and happiness either. We have to actively engage in it, using our intuitive wisdom and continue to walk towards our life well-lived. We are thriving in our third act because we work at it, we make it happen. We have made a commitment to sacred responsibility in our lives and Change-back Monsters, we see you! And we love you, and you are safe even though we have changed.

The bottom line is that at some point you will meet resistance. One of the reasons we aren't living our most authentic lives is that our families and communities have taught us to behave in ways that aren't right for us anymore. Many times they were not right for us from the start, *but* we hadn't made the time *yet* to get to know ourselves.

A big part of what makes our third act strong is the unflinching commitment to taking responsibility for the way we live. Taking responsibility for the care of our particular thread in the tapestry of our wisdom-filled lives. Let's face it, sisters, we have a lot of years of experience on our side and we know exactly what happiness feels like. We will not stand down when it comes to our lives well-lived, our legacy.

If you have ever pondered what your legacy will be once you leave this gorgeous green planet, know that your legacy will be the example you set by taking sacred responsibility for your happiness.

Honouring where others are

All of the people in our lives deserve compassion and love, as do you. Find your balance, actively engage your intuition and be honest about how others are affecting your energy levels and your happiness. You are meant to live your life, not theirs.

It is your Sacred Responsibility to Honour Your Intuition. You will know in your body and your heart when someone close to you is unable to have your best interest at heart. You have the wisdom and the kindness to shift that so that everyone understands the direction that will best serve a well-lived life. The more we put good data into the bank the more we write-over that less empowering data.

What data am I referring to? Remember that nervous ego that controls behavior? That ego is like a terrified creature constructed from moments when we were precious girls who didn't feel safe, loved and validated. Bad data is conscious and unconscious programming from when were little. We never chose this data. It was put into us so we could manage the lives we were given. As adult women we now get to choose the shiny and empowering data that goes into our personal data bank. And the more good stuff we pack in the less room there is for that old outdated stuff.

Are you aware when you are running off old data? It looks like "triggered" "jealous" "bitchy" "anxious" and talks with words like "should" and "can't. The more good data we give ourselves, the more we develop the courage to become an observer willing to stand tall and put on the brakes when old data is running our show. And in those moments when we are caught off guard and the old data takes hold, no big deal—own it sisters. "Sorry, I acted like such a jerk yesterday, I'll be honest— I was feeling jealous—oops old data."

Let's own these ridiculous moments. By owning them we bring them into the light. In the light we are given the capacity to hit delete—bye bye old data. The more we follow our passions and interests the more it becomes intolerable and impossible to live scared and small from that moldy programming. Filling ourselves with good data is fun and exciting.

The intuitive mind is a sacred gift and the rational mind is a faithful servant. We have created a society that honors the servant and has forgotten the gift.
—Albert Einstein

Our Fifth Sacred Practice

Our Daily Statement
Today I open myself fully to living a sacred life, I call in now the people, places and things that lift me up, light me up and hold me up as the accountable, responsible and authentic woman I am here to be. And so it is.

The Honour Your Intuition Imagination Practice (Imagining/Thoughts)

Relax your body, now take a nice deep breath in, and fully exhale.

Relax your jaw, relax the muscles behind your eyes, soften your brow and continue to breathe deeply. Let your cheekbones relax, let the roof of your mouth relax, let all the muscles of your scalp relax. Deepen your breathing.

Continue to relax your body from top to bottom, relaxing all of your muscles, bones, organs, and fluids.

Imagine yourself in the deepest state of full body conscious relaxation you have ever been in.

Now use your imagination and your detective skills to search each cell in your body until you find the one that holds the highest vibration of intuition.

Locate that one cell that seems like it's the brightest cell, the most vibrant cell, the most intuitive cell.

Gently scan your body for that one cell. It will reveal itself to you.

Breathe, imagine, and let this process unfold naturally and easily.

When you have located this single vibrant cell in your body, honour it, for its light and high vibration of intuition.

Take a few breaths and really honour this spark in your body, this original spark of your intuitive knowing.

Honour this light in you.

Imagine now as you focus on this one bright cell that you see how its light shines brightly on all of the cells around it.

In your imagination, you can see that those cells around that one cell are just as bright.

These cells are just as vibrant and fully vibrating with your incredible intuition.

As your focus expands, you see the cells around the second group also brightly lit with the highest vibration of your intuition.

You continue to see this bright light, an intuitive flow expanding through all of your cells originating from that first spark cell, the original seed of your intuition.

Imagining now, every cell in your body, fully lit up with the sacred light of your wise woman's intuition.

Remain here, relaxed and continue to connect with this full body imagination experience for as long as you like.

Breathing with the light and the intuitive force within you.

And so it is, you have restored your connection to the all-knowing light within you, your intuition.

**The Honour Your Intuition Breathing Practice
(Breathing/Words)**
Return to your Magical Moment breath.

Breathe, inhale, retain, exhale, and pause.

This breathing practice combines breath and imagination as we connect deeply to where our intuition resides in our body.

Imagine now, that as you inhale you are inhaling from the space between your eyebrows, your third eye.

Imagine drawing your breath from the third eye, right down into your solar plexus.

Use your imagination and follow your breath, follow it from your third eye as you inhale, all the way to your solar plexus.

Each exhale acts as a gentle exhaust system, relaxing you and releasing all that no longer serves your greater good.

Trust that your exhale is taking care of any tension, any holdings, any stress in your body. Trust your exhale and focus on your inhale.

Imagine inhaling from the third eye, pulling your breath right down into the solar plexus, into your gut, into the place in your body where you can feel your intuition resides.

Keep breathing in this pattern of inhale from your third eye chakra into your gut, and exhale tension and holdings from the body.

I imagine this breath in in the shape of half of a circle or a banana, one end at my third eye the other in my solar plexus.

The inhale comes in and follows the curve right to your

gut, to the place your instinct lies, to the place of "knowing" in your body. The physical expression of intuition where you feel what is right for you in your gut.

The exhale follows the curve back up and out, carrying with it any tension especially from your solar plexus.

Really focus on the flow of your breath and the imagination of the movement of your breath back and forth between the brow and the gut.

Continue to breathe and imagine this as a cleansing breath.

Imagine that as you allow yourself to exhale tension from the body, the exhale also takes with it any limiting beliefs that are clouding your pure connection to the divine intuition within you.

Imagine that this pattern of breathing is not only creating a deeper connection between your head and gut intuition but also a deeper understanding of the flow of that intuition throughout your entire body.

Your body always tells the truth.

The Honour Your Intuition Physical Practice (Physical/Actions)

Our physical practice is a series of eye exercises. It is said in yoga that we have our physical eyes and our spiritual eye. The third eye chakra is located between our eyes just slightly above our eyebrows. We honour our eyes, in connection to intuition, connecting to the flow of energy in this area of our body as well as giving our eyes and sight as much care as any other area of our body.

Rub your palms together, generating heat from the friction of rubbing your hands together, and when your palms are nice and warm, lay them over your eyes and allow your eyes to rest back in the darkness. Leave your palms over your eyes until the heat dissipates and fire them up again. Lay them over your eyes until the heat dissipates again. Do this one more time.

Close your eyes, then open and look up, look down, look up, look down, look up, look down. Close your eyes.

Open and look left, look right, look left, look right, look left, look right. Close your eyes.

Open and look top left, bottom right, top left, bottom right, top left, bottom right, top left, bottom right. Close your eyes.

Open and look top right, bottom left, top right, bottom left, top right, bottom left, top right, bottom left. Close your eyes.

Open and look top left, top right, bottom right, bottom left, top left, top right, bottom right, bottom left, top left, top right, bottom right, bottom left, top left, top right, bottom right, bottom left. Close your eyes.

Open and look top right, top left, bottom left, bottom right, top right, top left, bottom left, bottom right, top right, top left, bottom left, bottom right, top right, top left, bottom left, bottom right, top right, top left, bottom left, bottom right. Close your eyes.

Do each direction for 10–15 seconds to start and once you get the pattern down do them for as long or as short as you feel is good for you.

Chapter 6

The Sixth Sacred Responsibility: Create and Play

When we engage in what we are naturally suited to do, our work takes on the quality of play and it is play that stimulates creativity.

—Linda Naiman

Fun

Time and time again I see people turn down opportunities to play. It could be to try an instrument, or get out a few crayons and colour, to toss a coin in a cup, or any number of chances at creativity and fun, yet I see people simple refuse to play, and typically it is because they simply cannot bear to get it wrong.

Well, guess what folks, we can't get it wrong!

If we put crayon to paper or hand to instrument we simply cannot get it wrong when we experiment with our creativity. I'm not saying we will create a piece of art that blows us away on the first try, or even after the tenth try for that matter, but unless we start somewhere we will stay stuck in self-imposed limitations where creativity and play are lacking in our lives.

Any kind of expression of play or creativity will have the same effect on us so make it your own. If it is dance then dance, if it is music then sing or play. If it is sports then move your body, if it is writing then... well you get it. The Sixth Sacred Responsibility comes right after Honour Your Intuition, so we can be completely open to moving within that intuition toward our most natural expression of creativity and play. Getting creative and feeling that creativity as *fun* allows us to feel play manifesting in our life.

I am not saying each one of us has to take up painting or hula-hooping but what I am saying is get creative in any way that makes your heart sing. Start simple and begin to cultivate your creativity. Get creative in the way you plan your day, get creative in the way you make a salad, experiment with moving your body to music in different ways. Get creative by taking a different route to a place you go often. Pluck that crazy chin hair or grow it out! Just be the most playful expression of yourself and take sacred responsibility for your fun.

Being held back by our ego
Like all of the things in life that teach us, the ego has its place, many times as fast track to teaching us hard lessons. When we come at life from our perfectionist ego, too often we not only burnout, but we risk missing out on the joy of creativity and play. When we are in that part of our ego that demands we know how to master everything, or at least be an expert before we even try it, we miss out on getting things wrong. And getting things wrong at this stage of our game is not only fun but can be funny as hell. For me, that

in its self is worth trying something I know nothing about. I simply do not want to take myself that seriously all of the time especially when I am in a creative mode.

There is a National Institute for Play. Their mandate is "to be committed to bringing the unrealized knowledge, practices and benefits of play into public life. Gathering research from play scientists and practitioners, initiating projects to expand the clinical scientific knowledge of human play and translating this emerging body of knowledge into programs and resources which deliver the transformative power of play to all segments of society."

Limitations are self-imposed,
Take personal responsibility
—Marie Forlio

Founder, Dr. Stuart Brown has interviewed thousands of people to capture their play profiles. Yes, we all have a play profile! "His cataloguing of their profiles demonstrated the active presence of play in the accomplishments of the very successful. and the negative consequences that accumulate in a play-deprived life."

"A play deprived life." When I read this it really touched my heart. It is our sacred responsibility to play and we will no longer deprive ourselves of it.

NIFP teaches us about seven play types: Attunement play, Body Play & Movement, Object Play, Social Play, Imaginative and Pretend Play, Storytelling-Narrative Play, and Creative Play. We have no excuse to leave play out of our lives with all of these options presented to us by the very playful scientists involved in this research.

Body Play & Movement: The scientists say, "If you don't understand human movement, you won't really understand yourself or play." This speaks directly to the connection of play and our practice of moving our bodies. What may seem to an adult mind as "exercise" can be directly associated to play. So, raise your levels of joy. When you do your physical practice think of it as play, start to call it play and most importantly feel it as play.

They go on to tell us, "If you do understand human movement, you will reap the benefits of play in your body, personal life and work situations. Learning to play as an adult through our movement practice, teaches us about gravity, flexibility, adaptability and resilience. Play lights up our brain, setting the stage for learning as well as cultivating our ability to respond to the unexpected."

Object Play: Everyone loves to play with toys... Even a fiery and fabulous woman over fifty loves a well-made Hula Hoop™. In Object Play we are able to get the benefits of play with more than just toys in the traditional sense. But it is the attitude we have around play that will keep us tuned into object play. Give me a good mixed up sock drawer any rainy day and I am happy as a clam. Don't even tease me that you have a messy linen closet! Ahhhh... good times.

Social Play: This is play like "Tag" and skipping a jump rope, and the wrestling around of kids and animals at play. This way we activate each other in collaboration and creative response as well as interaction. I think we find tickle fights are in this category, too.

Imaginative and Pretend Play: In a rich practice of pretend play we continually cultivate satisfaction and creativity. The importance of this pattern of play, stands out for researchers when we are deprived of it. They have found that understanding and trusting others, as well as developing coping skills, depends on imaginative and pretend play. Knowing this piece of research highlights the importance of taking sacred responsibility for our imagination practices as if our happiness depends on it.

Storytelling-Narrative Play: Storytelling is found early on in childhood development and as adults we begin to enjoy both sides as story-teller and listener. There is lively joy and humor around how stories change in their description and truth as they are repeated. Enter the game broken telephone here! Stories invoke all states of feelings and in many ways, we nurture a story through telling it and it continues to thrive and grow.

Creative Play: This is our access to fantasy-play as well as to spontaneity. Here we plant the seeds for new ideas and fantasize or imagine all the ways they can grow. Use playfulness for innovation and a place to activate our amazing creative ideas.

All in all, find your personal method of play and get into it. Begin by seeing the activities you already love to do as play. If you love the activity it is not work, so it must be play! Start there and luxuriate in your enjoyment. The research is there, we simply must play.

The link to the NIFP research is in the resources section.

Create and Play and Sacred Sensuality

Sensuality is a gift for the woman in her third act. We have increased our ability to enjoy, to take pleasure in life and be unapologetic in our love for feeling good in our bodies. We have a natural connection as women to flow, to undulation, to curves, and to sway. This is quite different from our dear male counterparts who are gifted with a connection to angles, lines and a slightly more rigid way of moving in their bodies.

Women move in this sensual way by the nature of the female body. Tapping into how good that can feel ignites both play and creativity. Giving ourselves fiery and fabulous permission to feel unapologetically good in our bodies is our absolute right as a physical representation of the Divine Feminine life-force that moves through us. Our breathing practices are directly related to an honouring of this sensual life force within us. It is in the way we breathe, luxuriating in our breath, that invokes our sensual magnetism, activating and attracting creativity and playfulness.

Dr. Penny Kelly confirmed for me what I had already intuitively known and experienced in my life: being in a "turned on state" is one of the *best* ways to tap into higher levels of consciousness. (And, if you are not in the mood for conversations about 'higher levels of consciousness' I think we can interchange the words consciousness and creativity without losing the plot).

Our state of being "turned on" feeds our creativity and, in that, our ability to feel free to play. Penny tells us to get ourselves into a turned-on state and she says it with a huge smile on her face. She is fiery, fabulous, over seventy, and is one of my top five examples of women in their third act who mentor other women by living in Sensual, Creative Sacred Responsibility.

She also has observed that we are indeed moving into what she calls *higher frequency zones*. This means we must cultivate new behaviors to benefit fully from the higher frequency zones that are available to us. Most of us would agree that we want to operate from a higher consciousness and that we can access it from many directions. Putting ourselves into a turned-on state, where we are experiencing the pleasures of life fully, will activate our creativity, our ability to enjoy playfulness and light up the sensual nature of a woman of wisdom.

Being in a "turned on" state starts out as a practice, we build the new neural pathways to support this expanded state, and in time it becomes our way of life. And, ladies, once you tap into the pleasure of this sensual resource, there is no going back!

Tips for living in a turned-on state
Whatever floats your boat, ladies. You are the captain of your ship! Each one of us will find our own favorite ways to get us into a turned-on state. Here are a few examples from my own "play" book.

Self-massage with essential oils. Take your time when you massage yourself, this is not a mechanical process. Set the mood and luxuriate in your sensual self-care. Music— find your jam. Make a playlist of songs that make you feel empowered in your sensual, playful flow. Comfort, when you are home take responsibility for your comfort and how good you feel in your body. If it feels good wear it, and rock it! I'm a silk kimono and short shorts kinda gal. Drink out of your "good glasses", use the good dishes, and luxuriate in your Divine Feminine energy.

We cannot solve problems with the same thinking we used to create them. ~ Albert Einstein

This quote is great on many levels, but I have a particular interest in it because I think Mr. Einstein may well have been suggesting sacred responsibility! He says, "same thinking *we* used." *We used!* That is full and total responsibility for any problems created.

Sigh… it is all so intersecting to me. Yep, I confess, good conversations get me in a turned-on state.

The top five women in my life exemplifying this work are in alphabetical order because they are equal in the level of inspiration they provide to women and men world-wide. Learn these women's names, look them up and get totally turned on by how richly they love life, how inspiring they are, and how much vitality they have.

HeatherAsh Amara, Barbara Marx Hubbard, Jean Huston, Penny Kelly and Sue Regan Kenney.

Now go ahead and write down the name of a woman who inspires you to walk with that sultry, sensual, ignited feeling in your body, mind and heart. Then find another woman to tell about how this woman inspires you to "get it on" in life.

Our Sixth Sacred Practice

We Women share in the protocol practices with reverence for the potent possibilities that lie dormant within us. We accept our practice with open hearts and open minds in the knowing that these tiny acts of self-care grow quickly into a renewed love of our lives. We know in every cell of our gorgeous being that our practices fill us with the vibrancy of universal life-force.

Our Daily Statement

Today I open myself fully to living a sacred life, I call in now the people, places and things that lift me up, light me up and hold me up as the accountable, responsible and authentic woman I am here to be. And so it is.

The Create and Play Imagination Practice (Imagining/Thoughts)

Everything about our Create and Play practice has to do with flow, movement, spiral, sensuality, and the undulation of the figure 8, infinity.

Settle into a seated position for your Create and Play imagination exercise. Sit cross-legged on the floor or in a chair.

Sit tall and comfortably, balancing the weight of your head for greatest comfort in your neck.

Close your eyes and bring all your awareness to the base of your spine.

Begin to breathe deeply and easily. Feel relaxed yet strong as you sit.

Start to imagine now that your pelvis is a container for a brilliant ball of glowing energy.

It can be any colour and the colour can shift and change as you breathe.

Imagine you are observing this amazing container of energy you have in your body.

You notice how bright it is and how powerful if feels.

Continue breathing deeply.

Now with each inhale imagine you start to pull that energy up your spine.

The power of inhaling through your nostrils pulls this light energy up and around your spine.

Your inhales draw this light energy up and around your spine spiraling and spiraling.

Imagine you can feel its warmth.

Deepen your imagination and see this light energy split off into two streams that wrap around your spine.

Inhale, pulling the two streams of energy up from the brilliant ball of glowing energy.

Imagine your exhale acts as a gentle exhaust system, exhaling all that no longer serves your greater good.

Inhale and bring that spiral of energy up your spine and all the way out of the crown of your head.

Inhale, bring it up, exhale all that no longer serves you.

Imagine this energy as playful, creative light.

Spiraling and serving you, spiraling and serving you.

Maintain your focus and continue with this imagination practice for a full minute. Then as long as you like. But start with a fully focused minute.

The Create and Play Breathing Practice (Breathing/Words)

Stand or be seated for this breathing practice.

Level 1: Begin by breathing smooth, even breaths that are full on both the inhale and on the exhale.

Allow yourself to immerse into a hypnotic flow with your breath.

You are breathing as if your life is a sensual experience. Full breaths, in and out.

As you breathe deeply and easily, begin to let your body move with your breath.

Feel the expansion and the contraction as you inhale and exhale.

Breathe as if you are pulling into your body the most sensual music you have ever heard.

Begin to sway slightly, from side to side.

If you are standing, sway with your hips, if you are seated, sway with your chest.

As you breathe and sway, imagine yourself in a blissful flow with your creative life-force.

Go ahead and relax into your breath and into your movement a little more now.

Start to expand your sway and trace the figure 8 with your hips if standing, your chest if sitting.

Breathe and sway in the figure 8 for a minute in one direction, then shift directions for another minute.

Keep swaying in the figure 8 for as long as you feel moved to do so.

When you feel complete, sit or lie down and feel your body's response to your movements. Get still and feel the creative energy continue to flow.

Level 2: Play fabulous music while you do the Create and Play breathing practice.

The Create and Play Physical Practice (Physical/Actions)

Your physical practice to anchor your Create and Play Sacred Responsibility is a pulse of creative activation at the seat of your pelvic floor.

Using your exhale as your guide, on each exhale begin to lift the muscles of your pelvic floor.

Start by thinking of the Kegel exercise. (Mayo Clinic link to Kegels in the resource section.)

The muscles we are using for this pulse exercise are the same muscles you would engage to stop the flow of urine mid-stream.

Each exhale is connected to a pulse at the pelvic floor. Exhale and squeeze, exhale, squeeze.

Expand your squeeze to a pulse of three beats per exhale. Pulse, pulse, pulse.

Focus on the muscles you are squeezing, imagine with each pulse you ignite a creative spark.

This exercise helps to activate the energies in our bodies that have shifted from the creation of children to the creative expression of our authentic self.

Some of the physical benefits of this pulse exercise include strengthened muscles to support the bladder, providing less incidence of incontinence. Women with a stronger pelvic floor experience higher arousal and greater orgasm health!

Inhale deeply, luxuriously and exhale, lift your pelvic floor up and pulse, pulse relax.

Inhale, exhale, pulse, pulse, relax.

This exercise can be done any time of day. It can be done to increase your energy, your feeling of sensuality and to keep yourself connected to the creative energies that reside in the earthly energy centres in our fabulous body. Boom, chicka boom.

Chapter 7

THE SEVENTH SACRED RESPONSIBILITY: RELAX AND CELEBRATE

Well-being is making its way to you at all times. If you will relax and find a way to allow it, it will be your experience.
—Abraham (Esther Hicks)

Our seventh Sacred Responsibility is one that will keep us enjoying the journey. Everyone looks forward to relaxing and celebrating, right? You may have noticed that after reading this far, and participating in the Practices, that you have become more open to the idea of something different in your days. I know it seems simple enough. "Just relax," said the Lion to the Lamb. Just relax...

As we practice calling back our joy, and our time, we will need to be patient with ourselves as we continue to unravel our old programs. One of the most difficult and confusing areas of our lives is relaxing. As a yoga teacher, I have been watching people relax for over fifteen years now and I see how difficult it is for many to just surrender for even two minutes at the end of a yoga class. Yet it is the most effective way to reduce stress in our lives.

Yes, conscious relaxation will reduce stress for human beings. Unconscious relaxation will look more like watching shows that don't lift us up or having conversations that exhaust us instead of enriching us. These things do not equal relaxation but would be in the category of an addiction to stress if you do them repeatedly. It is something that will need gentle tending as you take sacred responsibility for your happiness.

Who am I kidding? Some of our stress-inducing choices may need to be pulled right out by their roots!

This brings us back to the absolute importance of acknowledging the gifts of a woman in her third act. Remember, way back at the beginning of this book, we accepted the fact that we are simply not needed in same ways we have been in the past which frees up our time and focus to do the things that bring us the most vitality.

We are talking about conscious relaxation here and it is no coincidence that it is lies in the position of our Seventh Sacred Responsibility. As we are rewiring our brain for radical happiness, we needed all the steps before this to be our foundation so that we may fully experience the freedom that comes with conscious relaxation.

Relaxation is indeed a game changer and we have the wisdom now to take the time to show the younger ones exactly how it's done. It is our sacred responsibility to relax, not just because we have some new-found hours of the day to fill with something and it may as well be relaxation, but because it is directly related to our Self-Care Practice.

Since we have tuned into the fact that making our happiness and our health is a priority, it only makes sense that we are responsible for a practice of relaxation. In conscious relaxation, we allow for the kind of rest that actually benefits our minds and bodies. This is an empowered relaxation. Our empowerment comes from the wisdom of our over fifty years on this earth and we no longer gain self-worth from rushing to multi-task our days away. We are empowered in our relaxation, we are empowered in our peace of mind and body.

I'm reminded of a time a few years back and being in a healing circle. In this particular experience, we would have long sessions of prayers, music and healing. I recall our Elder Teacher saying as he looked around the room at half of us sitting up while the other half were stretched out lying down and many dozing off to sleep. He said something to us like, "This is an example of how stressed we are in our day to day lives that we can't even tell the difference between relaxing and needing to sleep."

He went on to remind us that this is what it feels like to relax, and that it's doubtful that we need to fall asleep or even lie down.

I thought this was fascinating and I replayed what he had said many times over the years—checking in with myself around my true energy levels. I began to pay attention to allowing myself to relax while in a state of movement. I began to lower my shoulders from the position they had found themselves—up around my ears—and let myself relax and enjoy my tasks without any need at all to "look as if" I was "busy" to anyone. I began to luxuriate in taking my time, to savour the tasks and activities in my life that made up my days. I began to relax into who I am and the things that I enjoy. And it took practice.

Those of you who attend my yoga classes know quite well I like to ask the students what their energy levels are. I ask who has high energy and those who do raise their hands; who has moderate energy and those who do raise their hands; and who has low energy and those people raise their hands.

I have noticed that people typically do have a gauge of their energy levels. But more often than not, I see a handful of people who don't know what level of energy they have brought with them. Know yourself, expand your self-awareness and become clear on the ways you increase your energy and the ways you decrease your energy. Begin to understand what the state of relaxation feels like for you. We have years of fast paced stress-induced activities. We need to detox our minds, bodies, and hearts and conscious relaxing is a direct line to stress reduction.

The Fountain of Youth

I am going to just put this out there because it came to my mind in meditation and when it did a feeling of relaxation came over my body. It also felt intuitively correct.

I would like to propose that as modern-day women in our third act that we consider that conscious relaxation may very well be our fountain of youth.

Yes, our relaxation practice combined with our wisdom, combined with the desire to thrive, all collaborating to support us. Throughout history, people have been searching for the elusive fountain of youth. What if it was always in our reach? Our inner reach, yet we had been looking outside of ourselves all this time. If I am wrong on this one at least we will have fun doing the research. Ladies, I want you to help prove my hypothesis right!

Relaxing reduces stress of course, and we know that short-term stress can be helpful, but long-term stress is linked to many health conditions like frequent colds and infections, insomnia, impaired memory and learning, high blood pressure, hair loss, and stomach ulcers. Ladies listen up. Stress zaps our libido, and relaxation keeps us "in the mood"!

Being relaxed also helps us to make better decisions for ourselves. Let's keep this conversation going in our circle as we all delve deeper into this movement of a life well-lived, I want us to prove that relaxation is the actual fountain of youth we have all been searching for, so put on your lab coats, ladies, and start your research. Use your practices as your foundation of your research and let me know your results!

The Perfect Combination

Relax and Celebrate is a perfect combination for a sacred woman to end each day. I'm not saying to have a house full of friends over every night (and I'm not saying not to do that either) but what I am saying is a good part of the richness of life at this stage is relaxing and celebrating.

You have a life of so many amazing accomplishments, creative expressions and friendships to celebrate. It is important to celebrate these now that you have the time to reflect and remember the things you have done in your life—including standing beside someone else in their celebration. Yes, we celebrate others' accomplishments too, collaborating in celebration!

You may have come across gratitude practices on your journey that tell us to write down five things we are grateful for at the end of every day, and I love to do that. I also recommend we write down five things we have to celebrate as a daily practice. We will be discussing our gratitude further in the next chapter as we delve into the Eighth Sacred Responsibility. But while we are here in the Seventh Sacred Responsibility to Relax and Celebrate you will come to find that the Seventh and Eighth Sacred Responsibilities are constantly merging. A dance of gratitude, celebration and relaxation is more prominent in our lives than it has been in our past. It is more available to us as we have a renewed focus on what really matters to us. It is in the celebration where what is truly of value to us is exposed. We celebrate our past, present and future because all of life is a celebration.

Five Things I Celebrate Today.

1. _____
   _____
2. _____
   _____
3. _____
   _____
4. _____
   _____
5. _____
   _____

I inadvertently created a great new practice a few years back of waking up in the morning and the first thing I would do is call out, "Yay, we made it!"

You see, I had taken in a couple of elderly cats, a brother and sister named Arizona and Sedona who had been found in a less-than-beautiful situation. During their first year of living with me their age and health conditions became apparent. I found that Arizona had a form of cancer that made his wee bones terribly brittle and that he was in a lot of pain. It was his time to leave this earth and I was glad to have been able to provide a loving home for him in the final year of his life. Arizona was absolutely gorgeous, and I will post a photo of him on our group site for the cat lovers to admire. His sister and I, alone now, created a very sweet bond, and in my attempt to help her through her loneliness I started a morning celebration of being really excited to see her when I woke up and called out, "Yay! We made it! One more day!"

Even though I thought I was doing it for her, I found that I kept it up after she passed, and I still do it to this day. The new fluffy edition to my life, Phoenix, is much more aloof around my morning outburst but I love doing it and will continue my waking celebration happily each day.

Celebrations are what you decide they are. Moments and glimpses of appreciation for anything that made you smile. I can easily find myself celebrating almost anything. I had someone recently tell me, "you say thank you a lot." I was happy to hear that, even though I knew it wasn't meant as a compliment, but sometimes you just have to hear things the way that works best for you!

A sacred woman not only has a keen ability to celebrate herself, she celebrates others with an equal amount of enthusiasm. To truly dive into celebration as a sacred responsibility means that celebration is a natural part of your way of being. It means that you respect and celebrate life overall. If you haven't celebrated a full moon or a first snow fall yet, oh you will. This community of fiery celebrating women has so much to share with each other. Learning how each of you celebrate and what you are celebrating is one of my favourite parts of this work.

There is a huge conversation going on right now over social media and "fake" or "artificial" happiness posted in everyone's feeds. How we all seem to know that it is BS, that people are not being transparent and how seeing all the happy posts out there is making some people feel bad about their own lives, how they are lacking the frolic and glee that those on the internet seem to have found.

And for sure this is a conversation worth having. If you are so saddened by someone else's celebration it would benefit you to change that up for yourself because you are missing out on a free good time when you don't allow yourself to celebrate another person's joy.

We decide what activities are celebration worthy and if one of my friends wants to celebrate a cupcake with a bite out of it with a big icing grin then I would be crazy not to feel good when I see that photo. The cameras on our phones are amazing these days. At the right angle with the right lighting I could make the back side of a cat look worthy of celebration. (Great... now I have created a challenge for myself. Watch for more cat photos to be posted on our site. Yes... I am that person.)

Social media is just that, a mostly public, social community of every type of person with access to the internet. Some posts will speak to the inner activist in you, some with speak to the silly side of you, some will make you hit the heart button and some will make you delete but all can make you celebrate the fact that you are able to be connected to millions of people all over the world doing things that matter to them and letting you have a glimpse into a moment in their lives. And if you look at someone's happy post and think, "I know them, they aren't really that happy", then how about don't be their Change-back Monster. Let them eat cake!

Our Seventh Sacred Practice

Our Daily Statement

Today I open myself fully to living a sacred life, I call in now the people, places and things that lift me up, light me up and hold me up as the accountable, responsible and authentic woman I am here to be. And so it is.

The Relax and Celebrate Imagination Practice (Imagining/Thoughts)
A Celebration Award Ceremony!
   We begin grounding the Seventh Sacred Responsibility, Relax and Celebrate into our hearts with a huge celebration.
   Connect to your breath and allow a smile to come across your face, imagining yourself at an awards gala event.

Imagine hearing the hum and excitement of the crowded room.

You can hear glasses clinking as people toast each other in celebration.

Imagine yourself moving through the crowds of people saying hello and smiling. You know so many of these people and it is a grand celebration.

As you move through the crowds of people, you shake hands with some, greet others with hugs, and wave across the room as you recognize friends from the past.

You begin to notice how strong and comfortable you feel.

You notice yourself in a fabulous outfit in your favorite color, and you feel great.

It is time now for you to make your way to the stage.

This is your celebration ceremony and it is you who is giving out the awards to all the people who have been part of your growth in this life.

Imagine yourself now taking your place on stage at the podium.

You raise your glass and welcome everyone to the awards ceremony.

Imagine looking around and seeing how happy everyone is to be there.

The room is filled with every person you have connected with along your life's journey.

You notice how beautiful everyone looks, radiant and healthy.

There are people of all ages there and they represent all the time lines of your life.

You see teachers, friends, family, mentors.

You see people who have changed your life by simply having met them.

It is time now to give the first award.

You look at your long list and you call out the first name.

This award goes to_____ for playing a supporting role in my life.

Imagine handing over the golden statue or crystal trophy, or a plaque.

See yourself handing them their award, shaking their hand, hugging them with gratitude and sending them back into the crowd.

Your list and call out the next name.

This award goes to_____ for playing a supporting role in my life.

Imagine handing over the next trophy to this person, shaking their hand, thanking them, and hugging them with gratitude and sending them back into the crowd.

Calling out the next name on your list, then the next name, and the next name.

Imagine yourself continuing to handout these awards to all of the people from your life who have supported you, who have guided you, who believed in you.

Each award unique to that person.

Imagine yourself thanking every person for the award-winning roles played.

And be sure to hand out awards to those who have distracted you in this life, giving them the distraction award.

Give out an award to the people who have disappointed you, thank them for playing the leading role in a disappointment in your life. Shake their hand and hug them send them back into the crowd.

Continue giving out awards to everyone for everything that was brought into your life so that you could learn, grow, and change.

Give awards out to everyone who stood by you in your darkest days.

Give awards out to those who saw your light even when you could not see it yourself.

Give awards out to those who lied to you, as they taught you about truth.

Give awards out to those who tricked you, as they taught you about trust.

Get awards out to those who were inspired by you, as they taught you about leadership.

Give awards out to those who made you laugh so hard you could hardly breathe, as they taught you the feeling of freedom.

Give awards out to those who you have had the most fun with, as they taught you the meaning of life.

Continue giving out awards until everyone in the room has received one.

When your ceremony is complete, raise your glass, and toast everyone who has been part of your life. Thank them one final time, then cue the band to start the music. Imagine yourself spending the rest of the evening dancing up a storm with these award winners. Celebrate the rich tapestry of amazing award-winning people and experiences in your life for all of the wisdom they have brought to you.

**The Relax and Celebrate Breathing Practice
(Breathing/Words)**

With this breath to anchor Relaxation as a Sacred Responsibility we shift the breath pattern in our mind and begin with the exhale.

Still honouring all four parts of our breath.

Exhale, pause, inhale, retain.

Exhale, pause, inhale, retain.

Exhale, pause, inhale, retain.

Bring all of your focus to your breath and with your next exhale begin to follow the pattern

Exhale, pause, inhale, retain.

Say it in your mind.

Exhale, pause, inhale, retain.

Follow the pattern that has now shifted to focusing on beginning your breath on the exhale.

Exhale, pause, inhale, retain.

Stay focused on your shifted pattern of breathing for a full minute.

Then relax and tune in to how you are feeling and start again for another minute.

Take breaks if you feel ungrounded or dizzy.

This simple shift of mind set gives our breathing practice a whole new perspective to come from. Not only does it deepen our state of relaxation, but it helps to open our minds up to change, it shows us how easily and gently we can "flip the script", to change the stories we tell ourselves and to learn we are safe to write a new story for ourselves.

This particular breathing pattern brings about deep relaxation and can be used anytime of the day. It is extremely helpful to send us off into a deep sleep, kind of our own personal "counting sheep" exercise.

It is always funny to me how much coordination it actually takes to execute the new thought pattern as we breathe this way. Here we go, happily building new neuropathways in our brains!

The Relax and Celebrate Physical Practice (Physical/Actions)

Your Relax and Celebrate physical practice is to dance, so find a song or a piece of music and get ready to move. Dancing builds coordination, strength, and a sense of well-being increasing our range of motion and our ability to connect to our beautiful bodies. Studies show that frequent dancing improves memory and increases mental clarity. It has also been shown that people with Alzheimer's disease are able to remember forgotten memories when they dance to music that they used to know. Dancing helps keep our ability to think on our toes sharp as well as our ability to think ahead and plan. Dancing contributes to our feelings of happiness and experience of fun in our bodies.

We begin much like we did in the create and play exercise, and we sway.

Breathe and sway, then begin to add your arms.

Sway your hips, shake your booty and move your arms.

Experiment with moving fast and moving slowly.

Dance for one minute and then pause, breathe and notice how your body is responding to your movements.

Begin to sway, shake it, and get a little groovy.

For any of you fiery and fabulous sisters who are new to

dance I recommend checking out *Body Groove* with Misty Trippoli. She is one of my absolute favorite dance therapy instructors of all time! A link to her website is in the resource section.

Extra fun: I like to put on the radio and commit to dancing to the next song that comes on no matter what it is. This is usually pretty fun and many times hilarious. Don't judge the song, just dance to it, you may be surprised at how free spirited you actually are! Let this be a celebration of your body, a celebration of life and a celebration of your love for yourself. Listen ladies, we have nothing to lose by getting our groove on, and everything to gain. Get creative, get fancy, and get down and boogie!

A personal secret, I believe dancing heals everything, I have a pole in my living room.

A confession, I own four Hula Hoops™. Insert sassy winky face here.

You are so amazing sisters, be free in your bodies, enjoy your creative energy and move with love.

Your Personal Body Movement Secret _____

_____

Your Sassy Confession _____

_____

Chapter 8

THE EIGHTH SACRED RESPONSIBILITY: GRATITUDE

The best way to show my gratitude is to accept everything, even my problems, with joy.

—Mother Theresa

None of this will reach its full potential without Gratitude. Gratitude is the Eighth Sacred Responsibility and I consider this sacred responsibility a direct connection to our highest self, a connection to our full potential if you will.

Our authentic-self thrives when grateful. And the energy we are cultivating now of a life well lived, a life of thriving in our third act, ripples out to the great mystery as our full expression of who we are. We surf on the waves of the immense gratitude we have for this life and our position of empowerment!

The Eighth Sacred Responsibility is also your strongest ally enriching all the other Sacred Responsibilities, for without gratitude none of the other Sacred Responsibilities will shine in their full potential.

In Gratitude, everything has permission to exist.

It is funny to me what we complain about in our day-to-day life using words like I "have to" go to work, I "have to" do laundry, I "have to" clean the house. When we begin a life where gratitude is the prevailing wind we find our language changes and the emphasis in our tone is more like this "I am heading to work", or next level "I get to go to work today", "I am going to put a load of laundry in", "I'm going to put on some good music and clean the house today". I "get to" do groceries today and so on. We start to delete the complaint program that has been running for far too long and install a program of gratitude.

As intelligent, spirited human beings we have the ability to self-correct quite easily. Well ok, with a little practice. We can listen deeply to the thoughts in our mind and how we are talking to ourselves as well as the quality of these thoughts and in natural progression the quality of our words, then the quality of our actions.

I have discovered that it is my blessing to have clothes to wash, a job that fulfils me and little place to call home that I have the absolute honour to clean and care for. I have discovered that gratitude is common sense but not common practice for most. Sisters, we are not like most!

Gratitude and the wisdom teachings of the women who walked before us

As I wrote this book, I spent a lot of time in meditation asking for the most helpful words to come forward for the benefit of all of us women as we reclaim ourselves in the third act of our lives.

In this practice of getting quiet enough to hear my inner voice clearly, many unexpected things came to the surface, many of which I have shared through these pages. There was a continued underlying theme as I meditated: how much gratitude I had for all of the women who walked before me. All of the trailblazers, the activists, the suffragettes, the feminists, the women who taught us how to stand shoulder to shoulder with each other in the early Civil Rights movement.

Those who modeled what it looked like to never stand down in the face of adversity, the women who raised families as single parents by choice, and the women who paved the way to give us choice. The list of the women I have taken my lead from is long, and I am so grateful I found mentorship in their work. To the original fiery and fabulous women, I am deeply grateful to know your names. This book is dedicated to these women. If you missed the dedication at the beginning of the book, please go back and read the names of these women. Read their names out loud, look them up and learn their stories, then tell them.

My meditations brought me back to thoughts of the elders in our lives, the women who are the most seasoned of us, the women who are our mentors as we walk this path and my gratitude for the women who have forged the way for us to be as free as we are today. I also found thoughts of my own ancestors come to the surface and memories of life with them and their unique wisdom. During one of my meditations I had a memory come up of a time when my grandmother on my father's side, Rose Mines, chose two things she wanted me to have. One I will share here, the other I will save to share in person one day, so remember to ask me about the second gift.

The item she gave me was a piece of pottery. My grandmother (who I resemble a lot) passed on one of her most sacred items to me when I was 25 or 26 years old. It has taken me many years to truly understand the significance of what she gave me. Really, only recently as I found myself finding younger women in my life that I felt moved to pass down my own sacred items to, have I really tapped into the experience of receiving something from a woman in her third act, my grandmother.

I came to find that until I had reached a certain maturity myself I had not been able to fully receive the true nature of the exchange. Now as I find myself in a place to pass things on, I reflect on my own experience of receiving a treasure from an elder in the family. I now realize that the younger women in line to receive my accumulated treasures are also at a stage of maturing in the current act or phase of their lives and that it is a rite of passage for all of us.

I began to realize that the passing down of these items is not exactly what I thought it was when my grandmother gave me this particular treasure of hers. It was not simply that I "should" get this special thing because I was special, or I was the granddaughter, or that I was more important than someone else.

I see now she was handing down a feeling. She was handing down a story and a part of her life where she felt and most respected, honored and seen for the work she had done in this life, the work she was proud of. And she saw in me that I was the one to hold that memory for her.

Now back to the gift she gave me, the piece of pottery. I will freely admit that receiving this in my mid 20s was not much more than receiving a sweet gift from my grandmother. Grandmas do these things, right? But now I sit here in a different maturity and more able to feel the energy behind the gift she passed on to me.

The piece was a pottery basket and the handle of the basket was hand painted bulrushes. The basket/bowl was really more a candy dish that seemed representative of a grandmother to me at the time. But this was no ordinary candy dish. This piece of pottery represented the most important part my grandmother's life. It took my own aging and maturing to actually slow me down enough and take time for this memory to resurface to be enjoyed and to become a teaching for me to share.

You see my grandmother Rose had two sons, my father and his brother, and she also had two grandsons. Then there was me, her only granddaughter. So, it was simple for me to rationalize her giving me something that appeared a more appropriate gift for a woman than a man, and that line of thinking kept the pretty pottery candy dish in a certain category or compartment in my mind. As I matured my understanding of the gift matured also.

What my Grandmother was really passing down to me was an item that represented her self-respect and resilience. The respect she felt connected to her job, the job that allowed her to raise her family. She was not giving me her old candy dish at all, she was giving me something that represented the teaching of respect for self and how resilient woman are.

I didn't get that gift because I was the only female in the family, it was given to me as a physical representation of a story. The story of the richness of respect for ourselves and for one and other. The act of passing on an item to a younger person is rarely just to pass on some old dust collectors for a person in their third act, a person who is reflecting on what truly matters to them in life, but it is the handing down of a story, of their wisdom and passing the torch of that wisdom on to be shared through story and example by the ones gifted.

When my father was six months old, and his brother would have been about three, my grandfather went out for "a loaf of bread" and never came back. This would have been in 1947. My grandmother, now a single woman with two children and no explanation of where her husband had gone, was left to raise her family and work to support her boys—six months after the birth of her youngest son.

Needless to say, my grandmother had a lot of gratitude and respect for her working career as it was the very thing that saved her and her boys from a life that could have been very different.

She "retired" as an insurance underwriter with no warning, one day she went to work and by lunch time she was heading back home with a pottery candy dish. She was in such a state of shock that she had a heart attack after falling in the grocery store. A reminder to all of us that even the strongest of woman have vulnerable hearts, feelings, and it is an honour to know them.

I had many more years with my grandmother since her surprise retirement and her heart healing. She was a classy lady who made all of her own clothing and sewed designer labels into them. She held her head high at a time when it was uncommon to be a single parent and most certainly frowned upon by many to be a single woman.

When my grandmother passed away I had a female urge to go to her apartment before the men of the family did and clean out the more intimate places like the drawers with her underwear and bras and her personal care items. There was something about maintaining her privacy around her personal items I simply felt compelled to do and in one last story I received from my grandmother she taught me about loyalty and love.

In her top dresser drawer, wrapped in a stitched handkerchief, was a jewelry box with a hinged lid. I opened it up to see which of her many broaches was kept in there. To my surprise the box contained a corsage and a little flower shop gift card. A delicate and perfectly dried corsage and a note that said To Rose From Gordon. Gordon was my grandfather. That corsage would have been about 50 years old.

I was curious about what kind of support my grandmother would have had at that time and on the Government of Canada website I found out that she had entered the workforce as a single mother three years prior to the passing of the Fair Employment Practices Act and the Female Employees Fair Remuneration Act in Ontario, which was passed in 1951, and eight years prior to the Female Employees Equal Pay Act of 1956, which made wage discrimination based on sex against the law.

More currently, in a CBC News article interviewing Liberal MPP Marie-France Lalonde, dated April 1st, 2018,

Ms. Lalonde shares that after a two-year review of labour relations, gender-based pay gaps still exist.

Let me do the math for you, that would be 62 years *after* gender-based wage discrimination was made illegal. She goes on to say, "in certain sectors, part-time employees, (primarily women and new Canadians) were being asked to do the exact same work as a full-time employee but being paid minimum wage." In 2015 Statistics Canada informed us that Canadian women earned 87 cents an hour for every dollar earned by men.

Thank you, grandmother Rose for that candy dish brimming with the teachings of self-respect and for the powerful lesson of loyalty and love.

May we walk gentle, with a fierce fire burning bright in our hearts, may we walk in beauty together with gratitude towards peace and happiness. May we forever respect the gift of our life.

Our Daily Statement
Today I open myself fully to living a sacred life, I call in now the people, places and things that lift me up, light me up and hold me up as the accountable, responsible and authentic woman I am here to be. And so it is.

The Gratitude Imagination Practice
(Imagining/Thoughts)
Today is a day of gratitude and thanks to all the people, places, and things that lift us up, increase our vitality, have

provided positive reinforcement, and have helped to raise our consciousness.

You can never say 'thank you' too many times. You can never have the feeling of gratitude in your body for too long. Gratitude allows us to steep ourselves in a full body feeling that makes a magical connection with each other and the natural world.

When we allow ourselves to fully immerse in gratitude for someone or something that has been part of our growth, change, and personal expansion, there is an alchemy that happens where we create a high vibrational wave of energy that flows out into the lives of those around us as well as into the greater communities where we live.

This high vibrational wave moves further and further out touching other communities all over the globe. Gratitude has an ever-expanding reach that carries a sacred reciprocity that benefits both parties, as well as all who find themselves swimming in the waves of our gratitude.

Imagine yourself now completely relaxed with a huge smile on your face because today you are grateful for so much in your life.

We will choose a person, place, and thing and steep ourselves in full-body gratitude through our imagination and our ability to feel this gratitude in our bodies.

Gratitude as natural medicine
Imagine one person you have interacted with in the last few days for whom you are grateful. This is not a complicated exercise at all, quite the opposite actually. This person can be a friend, a family member, a teacher or someone that

held the door for you when you had your hands full. It can be a person who inspired you in a video you watched, you do not need to know them personally, you are simply recognizing your feelings of gratitude towards them. The feeling does not need to be associated with any details or action either.

And say to yourself, for one full minute while you imagine something like this:

"I'm grateful for the day. I'm grateful for the person who called to say hello today. I'm grateful for my eyes that see beauty. I'm grateful for my bed. I'm grateful for the moonlight, and so it goes.

I'm grateful for the safe travels of my students to class today. I'm grateful I have the opportunity to see my bestie today. I am grateful for how much my cat loves me. I am grateful for the view from my office window.

I am grateful for the fresh water in my taps. I am grateful I have meaningful work to do today. I am grateful for my friends who are into living a healthy happy lifestyle with me. I am grateful for this community. I am grateful for all of you who hold me accountable to this work. I am grateful for coffee, really grateful for coffee."

And so on.

Everything is fair game in this one. You are grateful for everything around you that comes into your consciousness *and* I like to add things like, "I am grateful for the things I have yet to learn. I am grateful for the things this moment teaches me. I am grateful for my experiences. Yes, I am grateful for it all and some days I am grateful for these tears that cleanse my heart."

Gratitude is the cherry on top of all of this. Gratitude is a game changer, it is simple, and it is 100% *free*!

The Gratitude Breathing Practice (Breathing/Words)

Connect with your Magical Moment breath.

Inhale, retain, exhale, pause.

Raise your arms to shoulder height and wide, open them like you are holding a huge ball.

Now imagine that ball is the Earth.

As you breathe, your arms open round, holding the Earth.

Inhale, imagining you and the Earth expand in breath together.

Exhale, imagining you and the Earth contract together.

Inhale expand, exhale, contract.

Start to feel yourself breathing in harmony with the breath of the Earth.

Inhale expand, exhale contract.

As you breathe, have gratitude for the whole of Mother Earth you hold in your arms.

Breathe and feel your kindness, gratitude and respect for the natural world grow as you breathe together. This connection and reminder to keep the connection is vital to our happiness and our health.

The practices of gratitude have the capacity to expand us to our next level of inner peace and connection to the creative force we all come from.

Be abundant with your gratitude.

The Gratitude Physical Practice
(Physical/Actions)

Our physical exercise anchoring the Eighth Sacred Responsibility: Gratitude into our bodies has two components. First, a meditation, and second, an action of a good deed.

Sit in a comfortable position, in a place that is free from distractions, especially computers and handheld devices. You are entering into a meditative experience of gratitude now, so prepare yourself in a way that honours the exercise. Get comfortable, focused and breathe.

Place your hands at your heart in prayer position, continue breathing smoothly and evenly as you allow the feeling of gratitude to wash over you.

Inhale, retain, exhale, pause.

Begin to whisper "thank you" to yourself, quietly aloud, or in your mind.

Thank You. Thank you. Thank You.

Thank yourself for being alive. Thank yourself for being so capable and bringing you to this place in your life. Thank yourself for being a caregiver to your body. Thank yourself for all your creative expression. Thank yourself for your success. Thank yourself for the wisdom learned.

Thank You. Thank you. Thank You.

Let your practice of giving thanks to yourself activate a sense of deep gratitude and appreciation for your life.

Stay with this meditation and continue to whisper, "thank you" and allow yourself to be showered in the vibration of your thoughts or words. Thank You. Thank you. Thank You.

Continue in the seated mediation for a full minute to start with and work your way up to sit as long as you can remain comfortable and undisturbed.

An added movement: keep your eyes closed and maintain this place of gratitude and thanks to yourself. Really feel it in the core of your body, feel this inner power of appreciation for all that you have experienced in this life, through your body, mind, and heart.

With your next inhale, raise your arms out to the sides and up over your head.

As you raise your arms up, imagine your hands can scoop up the gratitude energy you have created all around you while saying, "Thank You."

This energy of your gratitude that surrounds you gets scooped up each time you sweep your arms up on the inhale. As you exhale, follow through, use your imagination and bless yourself with this energy.

Inhale and reach up and scoop up the air full of Thank You all around you, and exhale, bring that energy to you and wash yourself with it.

Bring it down over your head and face, over your shoulders and body as if you are washing yourself with liquid energy.

Use your imagination as you add the movement, be as vivid in your mind with this as you can be.

Feel it, see it, imagine it, or simply pretend, all of these techniques work equally well. Choose which one you enjoy most.

Inhale, reach up, scooping the energy with your hands, now imagine you can press the energy of gratitude you have created right into your heart centre.

Press this liquid light energy into your heart, filling you with warmth and gratitude.

Keep breathing, scooping, and bathing in this liquid light of Thank You.

This meditation is designed to be done seated, yet it can be done standing as well. It works beautifully when standing in nature. Do this meditation in the forest, by water, even simply outside your front door or on your balcony or patio.

Spend as much time taking this in as you can hold the focus.

If your mind wanders, bring it back to Thank You. Thank You. Thank You. If you find your mind continues to wander and cannot be gently reined back in, then simply conclude the meditation, take a short break and come back to it if you'd like. This is all about you and thanks to yourself for keeping yourself alive and in continued experience in this life.

Go back to the mediation with hands at the heart and gently drop your chin to your chest.

Breathe and conclude when you feel complete.

Good Deeds, Selfless Service and Random Acts of Kindness

Our bonus actions for this Eighth Sacred Responsibility are contained in our second physical practice. Choose one and make it happen today.

As fiery and fabulous women over fifty, we are a force to be reckoned with in this area. We are wise, open-hearted, and loving—some of the best attributes to have in our tool box for just such a task!

Make a choice for this practice, choose either good deeds, selfless service or random acts of kindness and find a way to execute your love-filled plan. You can choose a category and allow the action to surprise you when the opportunity arises, or you can choose an action and see which category it ends up in after you have engaged in the action.

This practice can be done daily and repeatedly, and it is a practice that can be done in a group or as individuals. It can be covert, or it can be accompanied by a big band! The one common denominator with this practice is that we expect nothing in return for our action. We become stealth-like in our good deeds and we get in and out most times without being detected. For the record, International Good Deeds Day takes place in April each year, stay tuned for our community action.

Chapter 9

Maintaining Our Connection and The Sacred Circle.

Strengthening our Internal connection

Our first connection to maintain is always with ourselves. Following the 80/20 Rule for the Sacred Woman will help you to form a strong connection with your highest and best self.

The 80/20 rule was named by management consultant Joseph M. Juran after Italian economist Vilfredo Pareto who observed that 80% of our outcomes come from 20% of our inputs. (If you sit on any volunteer committees you may have noticed, 20% of the people do 80% of the work. It is funny because it is true!)

And this is where it gets real, ladies. When applied to living our sacred responsibilities lifestyle we can manage the expectations we have for ourselves more gently. If we now know that 20% of our efforts produce 80% of our results this gives us an exciting wisdom that is highly appropriate for a movement of fiery and fabulous women in our third act of life. We can have the knowledge that if we focus 20% of our efforts on thoughts, words and actions that increase our vitality we have a winning mindset, with the other 80% of our time being open to the great mystery allowing life to unfold and surprise us.

I know we are told to stop having expectations and we won't have disappointments. I love to challenge that in my life, just a little, because I'm sassy that way. I most certainly have high expectations of myself and I am also willing to be gentle with myself as I uphold them. And guess what! I am a fiery, resilient woman—a little disappointment now and again makes things interesting and tests my Sacred Superpowers! I also keep the expectations I have of myself narrowed down to just a few categories in my life. Eight categories to be exact, Self-Care, Rise and Shine, Know Yourself, Collaborate, Honour Your Intuition, Create and Play, Relax and Celebrate, and Gratitude. *And* I keep the 80/20 rule in mind when it comes to the expectations I have for myself in each of these areas. I do have an expectation for myself and all of you, that we be open to new perspectives that increase our vitality and our happiness. We can make change in our lives as much, or as little, as fast or as slow as we choose, but expect change. Be ready, resilient, and resourceful, sisters!

The truth about impulse
If we do not act on our impulse to do the practices, I believe a cosmic door slams shut. There is something that happens when we cut off our flow of inspiration and when we are inspired to move our body—we simply must. There are impulses or "messages" trying to speak to us, conspiring to move us.

I believe that this impulse is alive in the 20% and that is why it yields such abundant success, the 80% of benefit. Messages, impulses, nudges from our spirit helpers—whatever way it takes you to understand the power of the creative impulse, get to know that it exists in all of us and each impulse is a spark, igniting a fire.

If we do not respond to our impulse, the brain has the ability to give us the signals to do what we always do. By acting on our impulse to do the practice we begin to re-wire the communication pathways in our brain. We take advantage of the brain's neuroplasticity and its capability of stretching and expanding.

It is easy to think, "I don't have time today for that new thing I tried to start". Two days go by…then three…and we never got back to our simple Magical Moment breath and we totally forgot to play the pretend "I won the lottery game." The book is collecting dust by our bedside and we start to believe this was just another hope for a quick fix to change. You had an expectation of yourself and it is not looking like you had originally planned.

The reality is, you've got this, and we have got each other and sometimes we forget that we are making our own happiness a priority and that is absolutely ok. I promise, you will remember, and you will continue to build your life around your happiness becoming your priority.

The way to gently building our sustainable practice is one step at a time. Applying the Eight Sacred Responsibilities to an already transitioning life can seem awkward—like any new thing we bring into our lives. But if we introduce the new commitment to sacred responsibility gently, our rate of success and sustainability increases substantially. Begin by applying an effort of 20% in each of Sacred Responsibilities. You can break that down any way you like but I will give you a few examples as a template, taking Self-Care as our example.

I have a long list of things that make me happy in my category of self-care and I know I can't do all of them today, so I will pick one and commit to putting 20% more effort into that particular thing than I have done up until now. Breaking it down even further, if yoga is high on my list of things that make me happy and that is the piece I have chosen today I would increase something in my practice by 20%. It could be the length of time I move my body, it could be increasing my strength or flexibility by 20% it could be staying in that final relaxation pose for 20% longer then I normally do.

You could choose to drink 20% more water then you normally do, get 20% more sleep. You could practice your opera singing with 20% more focus then you have in the past. You may want to walk 20% faster or slower or further then you would normally walk. Which activity you chose know that the likelihood of a positive outcome can be found in the 80/20 rule.

I can break it down in time for you also. If I have a 20-minute morning yoga practice it would be logical that I would increase the benefits received if I added 20% to the time, effort, or focus. So, I can add *four* minutes to my practice and expect to receive an 80% return on my time.

The point of all of this is to make it clear that we are going to have great success with an extra 20% investment in ourselves. You can decide what the energy of that effort is each day. Whether it be 20% more physical effort, emotional or spiritual, every day you decide. Just follow your impulse and decide to do your practice.

Prove Me Right!

I have had this conversation going on in my heart for many years now and it is a conversation where we no longer put effort into proving each other wrong. It is here that I open myself up to all of you to prove me right on this. Begin to shift 20% of your thoughts, words or actions towards your practice of the Eight Sacred Responsibilities.

Move, breathe and imagine yourself living an inspired life that is sacred to you. Use our practices in some way each day as you increase your understanding and your diligence that a life riddled with happiness, creativity, relaxation, celebration and gratitude is yours for the receiving. Make a small step each day towards this becoming your new normal. The brain loves repetition, it loves routine, so give it that with our practices and what you will get in return is brand new pathways forged in the brain that support your well-lived life.

Nurturing our external connection

It is here where we begin the rest of the story. You fiery women are the ones to continue to walk towards what

You can tell who the strong women are. They are the ones you see building one another up instead of tearing each other down.
—Unknown

makes you most fulfilled. It is you who inspires other women to be the one who in turn inspires the next woman. It is you—fine, fine, friend—who keeps me accountable to this calling and I, too, will hold you lovingly accountable to living a life with your heart ablaze! May you forever be my muse and I be yours.

Our online community has a private place for group accountability, story-telling, support and celebration. Please join us if you have not already at www.reachyogalifestyle.ca

You can start planning your online Birthday party, too, because we are all coming to celebrate you!

This book is now your sacred companion. May it bring you deeper into a sacred life of freedom. It has been beautiful to stand beside you on this intimate and vulnerable journey of self-exploration. You have begun the practice and there is no stopping you now! What we are doing through this practice can very well be the new normal for the generations to follow. Where it is not only normal to have a "love your life attitude" but it is encouraged and modelled.

We've got this, sisters!

Now turn to the first page, and read it again, then again. Maintain your focus on your practices. Keep the interesting conversations going and continue to dream into reality your life well lived. Keep up with the research, because it is fascinating, just like you.

I love you all so much, thank you for joining me in this movement, it is no mistake we are all here at this particular time in our lives. This is the time when Fiery and Fabulous Women over 50 lead the way.

Rise and Shine, sisters. See you in the light!

Love,

Cathy

APPENDIX I

Chakra 101

This is a quick look at these energy centers, or energetic organs. I include their Sanskrit names in honour of the beautiful ancient teachings of yoga and the magical language of Sanskrit but please don't worry about needing to know how to pronounce their names in Sanskrit, just enjoy their beautiful names and relate to the chakras in the terms you understand best.

The Earthly Chakras
Our first three chakras, from the base of the spine to the solar plexus are our chakras related with matters of our Earthly life, while the upper three chakras relate to matters of our spiritual life. The Heart Chakra being the bridge between the Earthy and Spiritual worlds, but of course our heart is the great connecter!
* **First Chakra**: Root Chakra or Base Chakra called *Muladhara* is located at the base of our spine. It is our connection to the earth, our family, our tribe, relates to all of our basic needs of security and stability. When this chakra is in balance we feel safe, and free of fear

- **Second Chakra:** The sacral chakra called *Svadhistha-na* is located between the pubic bone and just below the bellybutton. It relates to our sexuality, our sensuality. Our creativity chakra is our creativity and sexual center. When this chakra is in balance we will feel alive, creative and free to really enjoy things like tastes, and touch, fragrance, visual beauty and music.
- **Third Chakra:** The solar plexus chakra is called *Manipura* chakra. It is located between our bellybutton and breastbone. It is also that place when you feel your gut sending you a message. I spoke of it previously as our personal power centre, relating to our self-esteem and will power. When this chakra is in balance we will feel like we have sufficient self-esteem in our life and a will to move forward in our lives.
- **Fourth Chakra:** The Heart Chakra called *Anahata* chakra is located at the heart center. It is the bridge between the energies of the Earthly chakras and Spiritual chakras connecting the upper and lower chakras. It is the place we relate to matters of the heart, love, forgiveness, compassion and connection. When this chakra is in balance we will feel ourselves give and receive love freely.

The Spiritual Chakras
- **Fifth Chakra:** Throat chakra called *Vishuddha* chakra is located at throat centre and connects us to our voice—to our sound, our song and all of the beautiful words that come out of our mouths. This is the place we speak our truth. When this chakra is in balance we

will feel at ease speaking our truth in ways of respect and kindness.

- **Sixth Chakra**: The third eye chakra called *Ajna* chakra, is located in the space between our eyebrows. It is where we relate to our intuition. We have our physical eyes and our spiritual eye. When this chakra is in balance we will see more clearly the bigger picture in our lives.
- **Seventh Chakra**: The crown chakra is called *Sahaswara* chakra or the "thousand petal lotus" chakra. This is where we connect to our higher self, to enlightenment and spiritual connection to all that is, creator, the divine. It is located at the crown of our head.

Note: The Heart Chakra has residence in both the Earthly realms and the Spiritual realms.

GRATITUDE AND ACKNOWLEDGEMENTS

To the Medicine Women, your support and interest in my light has infused me with a natural courage that is difficult to put words. A courage to trust in myself, but even more the courage to trust in others. To trust and thrive in collaboration with the natural world. Thank you for not settling for anything less from me then my realized, fierce, loving and authentic self. Thank you, Medicina, for showing me there is no separation between the natural world and humanity.

To my Soul Sister, Brenda, thank you for your unflinching dedication to our friendship. Your support for my life's journeys has been a sacred hoop, surrounding me with love and protection every step of the way. I can't thank you enough for *always* believing in me. For being my greatest flag waver. Mostly thank you for believing in my wild heart and always protecting my incessant need to *fly*!

To Kirsten, it is my absolute joy to be your friend. It has been my great blessing to have your fiery and fabulous heart ablaze with me on this project. It is your help, advice, editing and ass-kicking that pulled this book out of me. I am forever grateful that you have not turned your desk lamp off since this project began. If not for your belief in me, I would still be fumbling my way towards the finish line. Thank you.

To Carolyn, for keeping the Reach Yoga ship sailing straight while I was swimming in an ocean of pages. It can be a less than glamorous position being behind the scene and I'm humbled by your dedication to me, and our community. I see you, and I thank you for putting one of the original logs on the fire. Fasten your seatbelt!

To my Grandmothers, the original wild ones who taught me about what is possible. To my Mother, and all the women who raised me. I am fearless because I have followed your lead. Thank you for teaching me the love of music, dance, and importance of traveling to other lands. It is this that has taught me that home **is** indeed where the heart is. To my Father, for passing on to me the spirit of adventure and for setting an example of what loyalty to your life's partner looks like as an act of unconditional love.

To my deeply dedicated students, thank you for infusing my day-to-day life with incredible inspiration. Watching all of you rise and shine reminds me that my life's work has impact and reaches your hearts. May I continue to inspire you in happiness, health, and a love for this life! Namaste.

To the readers of this book, thank you for trusting your inner spark, the spark that made you pick up this book in the first place. Thank you for honouring your intuition and walking with me towards a life of Sacred Responsibility. Gratitude to all who have shared the practices and who have been inspired to live your wild, creative, authentic life.

I believe in you and your ability to rise and shine! May our path be blessed with an abundance of laughter, joy, and deep collaborations.

My final acknowledgment is to my teachers. If you have read this far, well, you are fully committed to my message in some way. As you read this allow it to flow through you and share in my words dedicating them to your teachers also. Even if you are unsure who they are for you in this moment just open to the gratitude and respect I have for my teachers. Know that if you have read this book you have benefited by my teachers as well.

To my fiery female teachers: Andrea Gutsche, Kahontak- was Diane Longboat, Groovinda Dasi, HeatherAsh Amara, Judy Uchikura, Lisa Couperus, Penny Kelly, Sue Kenney, Tracy Austin.

None of this would be possible without your love for me. Thank you for seeing me, and for not settling for anything less from me then my realized, fierce, loving, and authentic self. I bow to each of you in the depths of my gratitude and humility. May all that you have inspired in me come back to you tenfold. Thank you for pushing me out of the nest and always having a warm place for me to land. I hope I have not disappointed you.

Resources and References

Reach Yoga Lifestyle Website and link to join our online community. www.reachyogalifestyle.ca

Books
- *The Biology of Belief*, by Dr. Bruce Lipton
- *Warrior Goddess Training*, and
  The Seven Secrets to Healthy, Happy Relationships, by Heather Ash Amara
- *My Camino* and *How to Wear Bare Feet*, by Sue Kenney
- *Consciousness VOL 1. Consciousness and Multidimensionality*, and
  The Evolving Human, by Penny Kelly

Educators
Andrea Gutsche RPQ (Incredible resources on our Unconscious Mind a must read!)
- www.quantumintegrationprocess.com
Penny Kelly
- https://consciousnessonfire.com/
HeatherAsh Amara
- https://heatherashamara.com/

- hello@heatherashamara.com

Sue Kenney
- http://suekenney.ca/

Changing From the Inside Out
- http://www.drjoedispenza.com/

Kassia Gooding Holistic Nutrition
- www.kassiagooding.com

Barbara Marx Hubbard
- https://www.barbaramarxhubbard.com/

Jean Huston
- http://www.jeanhouston.com/

Ellen Eatough
- https://www.extatica.com/about/

Wim Hof
- https://www.wimhofmethod.com/

Heart Math
- http://www.heartmath.com

The Alignment Project
- http://thealignmentproject.ca/

The National Institute For Play
- http://www.nifplay.org/institute/about-us/

Articles

Heart Math Article in its entirety, a must read!
- https://www.heartmath.com/science/

Ordinary People Focus on the Outcome, Extraordinary People focus on the Process.
- https://theascent.pub/ordinary-people-focus-on-the-outcome-extraordinary-people-focus-on-the-process-6d9a0888df01

Neuroplasticity: The 10 Fundamentals of Rewiring Your

Brain, Debbie Hampton
- http://reset.me/story/neuroplasticity-the-10-funda-mentals-of-rewiring-your-brain/

Getting a good night's sleep:
- https://www.healthline.com/nutrition/17-tips-to-sleep-better# section3

Dr. Anne Marie Helmenstine PhD ThoughtCo:
- https://www.thoughtco.com/how-much-of-your-body-is-water-609406

Meet Your Happy Chemicals:
- https://www.psychologytoday.com/files/attach-ments/59029/happy-chemicals.pdf

Harvard Study
- https://www.inc.com/melanie-curtin/want-a-life-of-fulfillment-a-75-year-harvard-study-says-to-prioritize-this-one-t.html

Mayo Clinic Kegel Exercises
- https://www.mayoclinic.org/healthy-lifestyle/wom-ens-health/in-depth/kegel-exercises/art-20045283

Music and Dance
Medical Resonance Music Therapy
- www.scientificmusicmedicine.com

Misty Tripoli
- www.bodygroove.com

Rising Appalachia
- http://www.risingappalachia.com